Short & Simple Resistance Band Workouts for Seniors

Home Workouts for Mobility, Core Strength & Better Balance.

Marcherry Garner

Table of Contents

Get Your Free Access to All the Video Content

This book allows you to have **FREE access to our video course** where you'll see examples for all the exercises and workouts we discuss in the following pages. Throughout this book you'll see QR codes and links to the related videos. To be able to see them you'll need to register first.

The course is yours for free for life. Please take a minute and register now to get the most out of this book!

If you have any questions or issues with the video course please email us at hello@primelifepress.com.

Scan the QR Code or go to primelifepress.com/rb

Introduction

I have been deeply involved in the health and fitness community for many years, but I must be straightforward with you: my biggest reason for writing this book is pretty selfish.

I love helping people on their fitness journeys, I get a huge kick out of watching them succeed, change their lives, and do things that seem impossible. In all my years of doing this, it never gets old. My clients do, but the achievements don't.

My passion lies in helping the older population navigate aging with exercise. Exercise is the catalyst for many positive changes in their lives, and I believe it is the root of longevity. It offers you not only physical freedom but also impacts the social, emotional, and mental pillars of your life.

But it can be difficult as we age; I am well aware that the physical changes we are going through can be pretty challenging to navigate. This chapter is new and uncharted terrain for you, but I am here to guide you through it.

Whether you are just starting your exercise journey or coming back from an injury or time off of exercise, I want you to have the knowledge and confidence to face any physical health challenges with ease.

The exercises may sound simple, but do not be fooled; in their simplicity is their effectiveness. You will find a series of activities that will allow you to unlock your highest potential and help you achieve your fitness goals. They will be easy to grasp and simple to follow. You will be able to do all of these exercises from the comfort of your home and with minimal equipment.

Before we get into it, I want to applaud you for taking the initiative to regain your health and vitality, especially since the narrative in society around getting older and aging is so negative. We are fed these stories where we are the main characters who are set to lose physical and mental competence the older we get. It does not have to be this way. We can rewrite our stories and age with grace, strength, and independence.

I welcome the years to come, as it is a privilege to grow old. Not only are we wiser, but we also have formed deep relationships within our communities and families, We have lived through various historical moments, and we learned to know and love ourselves. We have been gifted full lives, and we can use the years ahead of us to continue to live with vitality and fullness.

But I do understand that we are frustrated. We are frustrated with the changes that may be occurring in our bodies. I know that I felt let down at times, scared, despondent, and angry. Suddenly reaching for a jar overhead on my kitchen shelf was just a little too difficult for my liking, and I found myself less sure on my feet.

Our bodies are going to go through changes, this is a fact of life. Our metabolisms will change, our bones and joints will get weaker, and we will find it harder to maintain or build muscle. We may notice a negative effect on our balance, and falls are more common among our friends. We may also notice a decline in our memories and find it harder to recall certain words; our moods may even change as we potentially become depressed.

As I said previously, this does not have to be our story. We do not have to accept this. I understand how difficult it might seem to be able to maintain a physical well-being in old age and as such, I am confident that I can show you how to work through this chapter in your life without the stress.

Many of the pillars of our lives will be affected; from the physical and the mental to the emotional. We are embarking on a very interesting time of our lives, and navigating it will be a test of all we have learned in life so far.

Exercise can have a positive effect on all these pillars. Yes, it will help you physically, but it will also help you handle the mental load that comes with aging as well as the emotional. Exercise has always been an outlet for me, and I am sure it will help you as well.

It may be a challenge at first, especially as a beginner, but I assure you the challenge of rebuilding your strength and improving your health is not as difficult as the alternative will be.

All we have to do is get started, and by picking up this book you have already begun your journey.

Inside Resistance Band Workouts for Seniors, you're going to learn about

- the unique challenges we face as we age.
- the importance of maintaining an active lifestyle.

- selecting appropriate exercises and resistance bands.
- the proper techniques to stay safe.
- how to modify exercises for specific body regions.
- exercises for improving balance and coordination.
- full body workouts for better mobility.
- how to improve alignment and flexibility
- full resistance band routines and workouts.
- advanced resistance band workouts.
- reps and sets recommendations.
- how to maintain a healthy and active lifestyle.

You can do this.

Tell yourself that you can.

Tell yourself that you are worth it.

All it takes is to get better by 1% each day. You have nothing to lose and years of longevity to gain.

Are you ready to learn effective and accessible exercise techniques to improve your strength, posture, and overall well-being despite getting older? Keep reading.

Chapter 1: Aging Gracefully

Life does not end at the end of our 20s, 30s, or 40s; it is continuing, and we need to embrace all that is still yet to come.

The role of fitness is to enhance the quality of life in these remaining years. It will play a pivotal role in ensuring that you age gracefully, with newfound strength, resilience, and joy that you never knew was possible. We all have the power to transform our lives, regardless of age.

Thanks to developments in medicine, health care, and an improvement in living conditions, we are living for longer than in previous years. But we need to differentiate between our lifespans versus our health span.

Our lifespan is the number of years that we live. Our health span is the number of years that we live in good health. It is the period of life when we are free from serious diseases (Peterson, 2017).

Therefore, it makes sense that we should focus on improving our health span to live out the rest of our lives in as good health as possible, and one way to do this is to exercise. Exercise, particularly exercise in later life, has been shown to extend our health span (Lieberman et al., 2021).

We seem to have the notion that as we get older we need to take things easier, slow down, and be careful. Where did this idea come from? I understand that as we get older certain mental and physical functions decline, but it seems that when we hit 65, we are considered old. As far as I am concerned, people do not just hit a certain age and get classified as old.

According to Richard (2019), there are three ways in which we can classify aging:

- chronologic age
- biologic age
- psychologic age

Chronologic age is your age in years and is based purely on time. It has little significance in terms of aging, but as we know, when we get older we become more susceptible to illness. It is an illness that causes decline, not aging itself.

Changes in the body are the criteria for biological age. Some people may be biologically old at 57, others at 70. Lifestyle and habits are two of the main influences on biological age. You can guarantee that exercise plays a major role here.

The final determinant of age is psychological age. This is how a person thinks and feels. My mother is psychologically younger than her age—she still goes out to local events, attends an exercise class, and has many hobbies.

So, you see, you decide when you get old, or at least you direct your journey.

Before we get into it, let's look at some of the things that happen to your body as the years go by and certain challenges they may bring.

Cells and Organs

Our cells and organs are aging. Cells get old and eventually die—this is a normal part of our lifecycle. There are various reasons why old cells die; they are programmed to do so, they have been damaged, there are too many of them, or they can no longer divide.

The decline of cell health means that the organs that are made up of them also decline in functionality. The testes, ovaries, kidneys, and liver are the organs that usually display marked signs of aging (Stefanacci, 2019).

Most functions usually remain adequate, but there is a risk that you become less adept at handling certain stressors. Organs such as the heart, brain, blood vessels, and kidneys usually battle the most under these circumstances.

Bones and Joints

As we age our bones begin to lose density, and we can develop osteopenia, or if severe, osteoporosis. This puts us at greater risk for fractures or breaks as our bones become weaker and more brittle.

Our cartilage will also begin to wear thin, which causes friction between the surfaces of our joints. The joints will not move as smoothly and may be more prone to injury. The degeneration of our joints can lead to osteoarthritis, which is one of the more common ailments in later life.

Along with our bones and joints, our ligaments also take on some wear and tear as we age. They become less elastic and are at risk of tearing more easily. The loss of elasticity results in a loss of flexibility and mobility and a weakening of tissue.

Body Composition and Muscle

At around 30 years of age, we see a loss in muscle mass and muscle strength. There are two factors at play here, the first being a drop in growth hormone and testosterone, which are responsible for building and maintaining muscle. The second is a decrease in activity. Between 10 and 15 % of muscle, deterioration will happen as a natural occurrence of aging but, according to Stefanacci (2019), any loss beyond 10 to 15% is preventable with regular exercise.

Eyesight, Hearing, and Smell

One of the first signs of aging is a change in eyesight. Depth perception, sensitivity to light, focus, color perception, and moisture incur changes the older we get.

We also may experience hearing loss, which may not solely be blamed on aging but on persistent exposure to loud noises over the years.

Our sense of taste and smell may also diminish once we hit our 50s, and we may find ourselves with a drier mouth.

Endocrine System

Hormones that are produced in the endocrine system may decrease, and their activity may decline. One of these hormones is growth hormone, which is responsible for maintaining and growing muscle. Additionally, insulin may become less effective and insulin production may slow down. This increases our risk of developing diabetes, a risk that we can lower by exercising and eating well.

Immune System

As we get older, the reactivity of our immune system slows down as the cells begin to react slowly to invasion from bacteria, viruses, and infecting microbes. The decline in the immune system results in an increase in the risk of developing cancer, as well as pneumonia and flu. The latter is more prone to causing death.

The Heart and Blood Vessels

As we get older, our heart and blood vessels begin to stiffen. The heart fills with blood more slowly and the stiff vessels are unable to expand, so our blood pressure rises.

Because our hearts cannot speed up or pump out as much blood as they can when we are younger, our athletic performance suffers. But the positive news is that regular athletic activities can counteract this.

Cognitive and Mental Health

Along with physical changes, you can expect some mental changes to occur as well. Short-term memory will decline, your reaction times become slower, and your problem-solving abilities will be reduced.

We are fortunate in that we have accumulated a lot of knowledge in our time, but the time that information is encoded, stored, and retrieved begins to slow down.

Other Challenges

Ageism

There are so many outdated stereotypes when it comes to aging that can lead to seclusion and discrimination in our communities. We may even begin to believe these ideas ourselves. Ageism and a loss of purpose are some of the biggest problems that elderly populations face, and these outdated ideas are not doing us any favors. My solution to counteract this? Turn to exercise as it can provide you with self-confidence and a renewed sense of purpose

Difficulty in Everyday Tasks

Losing my independence and ability to look after myself is one of my biggest fears. As we get older, and our bodies change, we may find everyday tasks more difficult than usual. This can have disastrous knock-on effects such as loss of interest in hobbies, socializing, and general self-care. This disinterest will age us much faster.

I truly believe that it does not have to be this way. By focusing on our fitness, strength, and mobility, we can ensure we keep our bodies capable of the tasks that lie ahead.

This is just one of the outdated stereotypes that are attached to aging—the idea we are not going to be able to manage by ourselves. We still have many years ahead of us that can be filled with vitality.

The Power of Fitness When You Are Older

Did you know that approximately 92% of older adults have at least one chronic condition, and 77% have two or more (American Psychological Association, 2021)? Along with these physical ailments, older adults also face additional lifestyle struggles such as loneliness, depression, and social isolation. These, although not related to morbidity or functional decline, still have a significant impact on quality of life and general health.

The combination of physical, social, and mental factors harms seniors' health and well-being.

Much research has been done on the impact of social and mental factors on physical health, and the link between the two has been proven extensively. Humans are social beings, and we need social interaction to lead fulfilling lives. A healthy social life has been shown to promote better health outcomes, while low social support, depression, loneliness, and anxiety were predictors of poor health outcomes (Hamar et al., 2013).

The older population is not moving enough. I strongly believe that movement is life, and research shows that movement in the form of exercise significantly impacts your life for the better. Lack of activity increases your risk for chronic disease and mental illness.

All that is required for positive health outcomes according to the Centers for Disease Control and Prevention (2022) is 150 minutes a week of moderate-intensity activity or 75 minutes of vigorous-intensity activity. You should couple this with two days of strength-based activity and balance-focused exercise.

You will see a marked improvement in your cardiovascular health and fitness, improved muscle tone, your bones will stay strong, daily activities will remain simple, it will be easier to maintain weight, reduce your risk for falls, and increase longevity. Plus, those who exercise also experience better mental health. The benefits are profound, and it is not too late to start and begin to reap the rewards that exercise brings.

It is a common trend that as we get older, we tend to exercise less, especially through the ages of 70–74 through age 85–89 (Hamar et al., 2013). By taking back our health and proactively working on reducing our health risk behaviors, we decrease our reduce or risk for morbidity and mortality from chronic disease.

There are not a lot of exercise programs that are easily available, you may also feel intimidated by the gym. This book is the perfect bridging tool to get you to your fitness goals. The exercises are easy to follow, they are designed for the senior population, and they can be performed with minimal equipment at home.

Remember, the only way we lose physical strength is because we stop using it. So how do you know if you are unfit or not? It's pretty simple actually—can you do simple everyday tasks with ease?

Ask yourself these two simple questions:

1. Does anything inhibit me from doing the things I want to do?
2. Is there a change in the way I perform activities that I used to perform before?

If you answered yes, then you should congratulate yourself because you are about to turn that around. If you answered no, then I applaud you for being so proactive and preempting any decline in your fitness. Here are the changes you are making to your health.

Maintain Independence

I already mentioned it, but this was one of the most motivating reasons for me to continue exercising—I wanted to retain my independence and not be a burden to anyone. Exercise keeps your bones, muscles, and joints strong, and it has a positive effect on cognitive functions. By keeping these two areas functioning optimally, you can keep a hold on your independence for longer.

Prevents Bone Loss

Exercise counteracts bone loss. As we age and our bone density decreases, we stand the risk of developing osteoporosis. Not only does it minimize bone loss, but resistance training has been shown to increase bone density when effectively used in a well-balanced workout program.

Maintains Muscle Mass

As we get older, it becomes more difficult to build muscle mass as well as maintain it. We lose muscle mass, and it becomes more difficult to maintain. According to Volpi et al. (2004), we lose muscle at a rate of 3–8% per decade after we reach 30 years old and after 60 the rate of decline increases further.

The loss of muscle mass is one of the major causes of disability and loss of independence amongst the older population, as it makes the risk of falls and major injury rise.

The loss of muscle mass also affects body composition, as we see a rise in body fat as we get older. The increase in body fat may trigger insulin resistance, which in turn can have implications for type 2 diabetes, obesity, heart disease, and osteoporosis.

Relieves Aches and Pains

It may seem contrary to what you might expect, but exercise can reduce aches and pain, especially the pain and stiffness that is associated with arthritis. By strengthening the muscles around your joints, you take the pressure off them and relieve the stress. The movement also reduces inflammation and makes the joints more mobile (National Council On Aging, 2021).

Helps Prevent Chronic Disease

As we age we are more susceptible to developing chronic diseases such as diabetes, cardiovascular disease, cancer, obesity, and hypertension. Exercise is a tool we can use to minimize our risks of falling ill with any of these ailments.

For those who already suffer from chronic illness, exercise can help alleviate the symptoms and help them lead a better quality of life.

The beneficial effects of working out also extend past the physical to the cognitive, with studies showing that exercise has positive benefits in the fight against cognitive decline. It seems that by exercising consistently, you can slow the progress of Alzheimer's in those at risk (Okonkwo, 2019).

Improves Mental Health

Exercise releases endorphins, which are hormones that make us feel good. It can help alleviate anxiety and depression as well as reduce stress. Exercise also makes us more self-confident and improves our self-esteem. This adds to our overall sense of well-being, which is important for anyone, regardless of age.

The connection between physical health and mental well-being cannot be denied, and the nurturing of our mental health should be just as big a priority to exercise as maintaining our physical fitness is.

The changes to our mental health, as we get older, can be just as profound as the changes to our physical health, and I am pleased that mental health awareness is becoming a more common topic and focus.

Forms a Keystone Habit

Your exercise routine could help you maintain other healthy habits that will benefit your well-being. It has been shown that by keeping up an exercise routine you are more likely to maintain habits such as eating well, sleeping well, and managing your stress. These knock-on effects create a well-balanced and healthy lifestyle that is easy to maintain

Improves Sleep

Sleep is very important for health and allows 0ur body and mind to recover and reset. As we get older, we may experience sleep disturbances and find it difficult to get the quality sleep that we need.

Exercise can help you fall asleep, get better quality sleep, and wake up more energized and refreshed for the day.

Myths About Exercise

I understand that starting or maintaining an exercise routine can be hard. In addition to aches, pains, and various health problems, you may also have many additional concerns about exercising as a senior stemming from what you may have heard online or via others.

I want to make sure that you have the right information and that you are not believing any unfounded myths about exercising as an older person.

You may feel that it is too late for you to start exercising and that you are too old for it to have any benefit. You may also feel nostalgia for what you were capable of when younger and feel it is now just a waste of time.

This is exactly why you should start moving and exercising again! You have read through the list of benefits and know that exercise at any age can only bring positive results. There is no need for you to have to slow down and take it easy as you get older. If you want to live a life full of energy, vitality, and adventure, you will need to maintain a certain level of fitness.

And remember, it does not require hours at the gym or on the treadmill. All it takes is a resistance band and some clear floor space in your home. Let's look at the self-talk that could be holding you back.

Exercise Is Pointless, I am Going to Age Anyway

Yes, you are aging, but exercise can soften the physical and mental effects that arise when getting old. It can help you feel younger and be a powerful tool for retaining your independence as you get older.

I Am too Old to Start

This is one of the biggest misconceptions when it comes to fitness. You are never too old to reap the benefits of exercise. All you have to do is start where you are and gradually build up your capacity. The physical and mental rewards will be well worth it, and you will feel the difference almost immediately.

Exercise Is Risky and I May Get Injured

You should always get the all-clear from your doctor before you begin any exercise routine, this should put your mind at ease. Additionally, if you are following a well-thought-out exercise program that takes into consideration your individual needs, your likelihood of injury is low.

As you know, exercise builds strength and physical capacity and these make you more physically capable, thus reducing your chances of injury or falls.

If you do injure yourself (whether it is during exercise or daily life) having a strong body from previously working out will help you heal faster.

I Will Never Be Capable of What I Once Was

Our capabilities as we get older are inevitably affected due to the changes in hormones, muscle mass, bone density, and metabolism. But you should still be very proud of your physical achievements regardless of what they may look like, not many people take their health and well-being seriously, especially as they get older. Your physical investment is something to be celebrated.

Take some time to set appropriate goals when it comes to your fitness and watch how successfully you can reach them. It is also important to realize that by choosing to be less active, you are doing more damage to your fitness than aging ever would.

I Cannot Exercise Because I Am Disabled

If you are limited from performing certain movements because you are chair-bound, there are a variety of exercises that can be performed in a chair. Some of the exercises in this book can be modified and used to build strength and improve muscle tone, flexibility, and mobility.

I Have Too Many Aches and Pains

At the risk of sounding like a stuck record and repeating myself—exercise can help! When you start moving, not only do you improve your strength, but you also can relieve any niggles and sore spots you may have. Plus, it gives your self-confidence a boost. Many of my clients, before starting exercise, felt weak and thought they did not have the physical strength or fitness to start exercising. All it took was one to two weeks of consistent resistance band workouts to begin to feel stronger, more capable, and more confident in their bodies.

The Cost of Joining a Gym Is too Expensive

Gym memberships can be expensive, but the great thing about this book is that it provides you with exercises and workouts that you can do from the comfort of your home and with minimal equipment.

This book is all you will need, and you will be able to save on commuting costs and membership fees. Plus working out from home offers you more convenience and lets you save time, you are also more likely to work out if it is easier to do so, and what could be easier than working out from your bedroom or lounge?

I Have no Time

Even 10 or 20 minutes of exercise a day can give you benefits and increase your health and wellness. You do not need hours in the gym, this book provides you with simple and easy workouts you can do in the comfort of your home whenever you find some time.

It is your responsibility to make exercise a priority and even though we live quite frantic lives, there is a way you can squeeze in some time to work on your health. Whether it is 10 minutes a day during the week and then longer sessions over the weekend, with some dedication and motivation you can get it done.

I Am too Tired

Great! Exercise can help as it provides you with more energy. This may seem counterintuitive, but exercise can reduce fatigue, increase alertness, and improve your focus.

The Benefits of Resistance Band Training

Resistance bands are a popular workout tool for several reasons including convenience, affordability, adaptability, and portability. This makes them a home gym must-have.

These bands are either fabric or elastic and add tension and resistance to movements to increase their difficulty and engage your muscles to work harder, thus building and maintaining strength.

Resistance bands offer a great workout for both beginners and more advanced athletes. They are incredibly versatile and come in a range of different resistances, from light to heavy. They are also a safe and gentle way to exercise and provide low-impact stimulus.

Variety

There are no limits to the type of exercise you can do with a resistance band. From strength training and stretching to balance and mobility-focused exercises, resistance bands are a must piece of equipment that gives you great returns.

You can work for almost every muscle group and get a full-body workout. They are efficient at targeting our larger muscles and also build strength in our smaller supporting muscles. This leads to many physical benefits such as strengthening your core, back, and shoulders, which in turn help your stability and posture (Biddulph, 2021).

Versatility

Resistance bands are very versatile. The majority of things that you can do with a weight you can do with a resistance band. From bicep curls to good mornings, resistance bands can be utilized in creative ways to get the workout you need.

Easy to transport, they are great to take on holiday, and they are affordable as well.

Provides a Full-Body Workout

A band that provides stronger resistance will be used to work your bigger muscles such as glutes and thighs. The lighter bands can be used to work your smaller muscles such as your shoulders, upper back, and calves. They can also be used for stretching and mobility exercises.

Bands are often unstable, and this element of tension creates a more challenging workout than if you were to use free weights such as a kettlebell or dumbbell. Additionally, you can do a wide variety of compound movements with them, which ensures a full-body workout that makes you more efficient and reduces your time spent working out.

You are in control of the amount of resistance you use when working out, so each movement is 100% adaptable to your fitness level and can be modified as such.

Increases Time Under Tension

Time under tension refers to how long your muscles spend exercising force to perform a movement.

For example, if you perform a bodyweight squat, your leg muscles are more challenged when they raise your body out of the squat into a standing position.

If you place a resistance band around your shoulders and under your feet, you make the movement more difficult as your legs fight the additional resistance of the band. Additionally, with the addition of the band, your legs need to fight the downward pull as well.

This requires additional tension from your muscles through both stages of the movement: the downward phase and the upward phase.

Burns Fat

Exercises that incorporate resistance work are great for aiding in fat loss. Resistance exercises create a post-workout caloric burn, which is referred to as excess postexercise oxygen consumption or EPOC (Head, 2021). In simple terms, this is the energy used by your body once it has completed exercising and is beginning to recover and turn back into its pre-workout state.

Resistance band exercises, unlike cardio, build and maintain muscle mass. The more muscle mass we have, the more calories we burn at rest. Muscle uses a lot of calories to maintain, so by just having muscle, our metabolic rate is significantly higher than without it.

Improves Mobility

Wear and tear of our joints, bones, cartilage, and muscles is bound to occur as we get older. We can stave this off by continuing to be active and moving more throughout the day, as well as partaking in a well-designed exercise program that incorporates stretching and balance exercises.

When added to a routine stretching exercise, resistance bands can amplify the stretch and make it more challenging if needed. They can be used to gently increase your range of motion as you progress through each movement and need to challenge yourself more.

Improves Posture and Relieves Aches

Working out allows you to connect with your body and creates better body awareness. This can translate into better posture as you become more aware of how your body moves and how you hold yourself in relation to your environment.

By learning about and improving your posture, you can alleviate some of the aches and pains you may be feeling that are caused by placing your body in non-ideal positions.

Reduces Risk of Injury

Resistance bands are beginner-friendly and easy to learn how to use with good form. They are low-impact so even though they provide the same type of stimulus to your muscles, they do so in a way that lowers the amount of force on your joints (Pinkham, n.d.).

This is particularly beneficial to those who may be suffering from arthritis and experiencing joint pain.

Resistance bands also promote good form and movement patterns. I have often seen clients, when tired, use momentum to complete a movement or move a weight. When presented with a band, you cannot use any external force but your strength to complete the movement. This promotes correct and safe movement patterns and allows you to only complete what you are physically capable of.

Key Takeaways

Resistance bands may not be the sexiest piece of workout equipment in a gym or at home, but they are effective and provide an exercise stimulus that will get you results, whether that is purely functional or aesthetic.

This unassuming exercise tool is portable, versatile, affordable, and easy to use. They can be used to modify any exercise to suit any fitness level, they can be paired with any other piece of gym equipment, and they are safe.

Free weights, barbells, and bumper plates along with resistance bands all have their place in your exercise routine but for us, at this stage on our fitness journeys, resistance bands are the perfect tool to accelerate us towards wellness.

There have been numerous studies conducted amongst older populations and their incorporation of resistance bands into their workout routines, and the results were very compelling.

According to Smith et al. (n.d.) after placing their older participants in an eight-week-long resistance band exercise program they saw an increase in their leg strength and flexibility, pain and fatigue, blood vessel dilation, and improvement in general health.

Studies by Ponce-Bravo et al. (2015) showed an increase in gross motor skills, grip, and arm strength. Participants also showed improved reaction times.

Finally, if you are a postmenopausal woman you may benefit from improved insulin, glucose, and blood lipid profiles which reduces the risk of cardiovascular disease (Son & Park, 2021).

Now that we are aware of all the benefits of this training method, let's get started on our journey.

Chapter 2: Getting Started

The following chapter will prepare you to start working out safely and effectively. I spent the majority of this book highlighting the benefits of working out and why you should be incorporating it into your daily life, but taking action and making it a consistent habit may take a little bit of effort and motivation.

We will discuss health considerations, space, and equipment, warm-ups and cooldowns, ways to make the "habit" stick as well as any other bits of advice I can provide to make this part of your health journey as easy as possible.

Consult With Your Healthcare Provider

Regardless of whether you are new to exercise, returning after some time off, or seasoned in the gym, you must talk to your healthcare provider before beginning any new exercise regime.

Although moderate physical exercise is recommended for most people, you do need to make sure that you get a thorough physical exam before beginning to work out. This is to confirm that to ensure that you have no underlying conditions that may limit your exercise options.

If you have or had any injuries, these may also impact the kind of exercise you do or limit certain movements that you may be able to perform. This screening process will guide you in creating an individualized exercise plan that will complement your current health and fitness levels. For example, your doctor may advise that you work out more or less depending on your current health status.

Make sure that you bring up any of the following topics when visiting your doctor:

- Your current exercise routine or lack thereof. Discuss how often and what kind of exercise you currently do.
- Your current medical issues such as high blood pressure, arthritis, asthma, or diabetes for example.
- You have undergone any surgical procedures.
- You are under medical supervision for a condition.

If you have been given the go-ahead to exercise, there are some situations where you should contact your doctor.

- Any shortness of breath, dizziness, or lightheadedness.
- Rapid heartbeat.
- Numbness or pain in your joints or muscles that lasts for a prolonged period.
- Lower leg or back pain that lasts even during rest.
- Headaches during or after exercise.

Remember to always listen to your body and know when to push and when to hold back and ease off.

Set Goals and Plan Your Path

Take some time to set some goals. Grab a notebook and pen or use your notes app on your phone and think about what you want to achieve and write it down.

I suggest that in the beginning, you think of short-term goals that can be achieved fairly easily. As your fitness level grows, so can your goals. By choosing goals that you are sure to accomplish albeit with some hard work, you will feel a sense of accomplishment, and pride and increase your confidence. This will keep you motivated to strive to accomplish more as you steadily tick off your goals.

A simple place to start is to set the goal of doing two workouts a week. That is usually where I start my clients off, it also eases them into their workout routine without the risk of taking too much on and potentially burning out or injuring themselves.

A great and quite popular goal-setting formula is known as the S.M.A.R.T method.

- specific
- measurable
- achievable
- relevant
- time-bound

Specific

Reflect on your goal and describe it as specifically as possible. To double down and focus, it needs to be clear and provide motivation.

As you sit down and write down your goal, ask yourself why you have set it and what it is its importance to you. Consider the resources you have to accomplish it.

Put your goal somewhere where you can see it often as a reminder of what you are working towards.

Example: *I want to work out two times a week so that I can get stronger to confidently go hiking with my children on the weekends.*

Measurable

You should be able to track your progress to stay accountable and keep you motivated. You will also be able to evaluate and adjust your plan if necessary if you find you are not on track.

Tracking your progress keeps you motivated, focused, and excited.

Example: *After six weeks of a consistent exercise routine, I want to add a workout day.*

Achievable

Your goal should be attainable but should also be difficult enough to challenge you, so you have to put in the effort.

Before setting your goal, evaluate how achievable it is given any constraints you may have. Are there any financial, timing, or health considerations to take into account?

Example: *My current fitness levels allow me to do two workouts a week. When I get fitter, I can add a third.*

Relevant

Not only should your goal matter to you, but it should also complement or relate to any other goals you may have.

Ask yourself if your goal is worthwhile. Is it the right time for you to be undertaking it? How does it affect the other areas of your life?

Example: *Exercise will help me lead a more fulfilling active life. There is no time like the present.*

Time-Bound

As you plan your goal, it is important that you set up milestones for yourself, so you can have something to work towards. This allows you to keep focus on your goal and motivates you to do something every day or every week to accomplish it.

Within what time do you want to reach this goal? What can you do today to help get you closer to achieving it? What can you do this week? What can you do this month?

Example: Tonight I can put out my exercise clothing and shoes so that it is ready for me to get into tomorrow morning.

Track Your Progress

Use a notebook or phone app to track your workouts and your progress. Every week, write down your routine and log how many sets and reps you did, as well as the resistance band that you used.

This is important data that will let you know how to structure the rest of your program and how to progress and get stronger. This allows you to make any adjustments if needed and lets you know how your body is responding to the increased activity.

Workout tracking is also a good way to keep motivated. Each week you will have proof that you are getting stronger, fitter, and healthier, which will incentivize you to keep up your routine.

Keep accountable, motivated, and confident by simply keeping track of your workouts—it takes five minutes and brings plenty of useful insight.

Create a Routine

Consistency will get you results. By exercising regularly and turning your routine into a habit that you tick off every week, you have a greater chance of sticking to it and reaching your goal.

There are several ways to make a habit stick. One is to replace a bad habit with a good one. You can choose to swap 30 minutes of television for exercise.

You could also create a habit and routine by working out at the same time every day. For example, you could exercise after breakfast every morning and get it done by the start of the day. Choose a time that works best for you and that you can stick to.

Go Easy on Yourself

There are some times when you may miss a workout or not feel up to it. Give yourself some grace and just pick up where you left off. You mustn't hold onto an all-or-nothing mindset. Each choice you make, from taking a walk to eating more vegetables, to working out counts and adds up to a successful day of health.

On the days that you feel tired or not up to working out, get dressed and commit to starting the warm-up only. Gauge how you feel after doing that—the chances are you will get into it and continue. Alternatively, relook at your exercise program and switch things up if you need something more "fun" to do to get you motivated for that particular session.

Automate Your Habit

A trigger is an event that will set off an alternative event. So when A happens, B will follow; they are simple reminders that are like a cue, time of day, or particular action.

These triggers let you complete tasks as if you were on autopilot, like brushing your teeth after breakfast or drinking a glass of water when you wake up.

Find a trigger (or create one) that can lead into your exercise routine. I usually have a banana or some fruit around 1 p.m. as a pre-workout snack, which triggers me into doing my workout that afternoon.

Reward Yourself

Of course, long-term rewards such as good sleep, improved health, an increase in energy, and improvement in mood are strong motivators for exercising, but in the beginning, it may be a good idea to give yourself some smaller incentives.

Simple things such as treating yourself to a delicious post-workout cup of coffee, smoothie, long bath, or even new workout gear can help motivate and encourage you to follow through with your exercise routine. The key is to only allow yourself the reward after exercise.

Hold Yourself Accountable

Let your friends and family members know what you are trying to achieve and ask them to check in on you. Accountability is a great tool for keeping us on the path to our goals as not only does it make us more responsible for our actions but it also gives us more motivation to reach them as there are now people counting on us to stick to our word.

Let your friends, family, and even your doctor know what your plans are and keep them updated with your progress, or approach them for help when you need an extra bit of motivation and support.

Setting Up Your Space

You do not need a lot of space for your new home gym. If you do have a lot of area to work with, that is great, but the benefit of this kind of training is that you can do it anywhere as long as you have your bands on you.

Use the information provided to create the space you are capable of creating. It will help motivate and encourage you to work out if you have a designated area for exercise, regardless of what that may look like for you.

Find the Right Area in Your Home

Whether you have a spare room, garage, or the corner of your dining room or lounge—you can use any space available to create an exercise haven for yourself.

Once you have chosen an area, decide how you will set it apart from the rest of the house. I laid down some flooring and mats in our garage to protect the floor.

You do not have to do the same, but for me, I needed a clear separation between my living space and my exercise space. This separation of spaces also meant that I was less distracted during my workouts and could be present with what I was doing.

Gather Your Equipment

Realistically, all you require is your body and your resistance bands, but there are some movements that you can or may need to perform in a chair. Some basics you should add to your gym setup are:

- your resistance bands

- storage boxes
- a comfortable chair or bench
- a yoga mat
- a towel
- a skipping rope for warm-ups
- a fan
- notebook and paper

These are the basics and can be simplified even further as well. You can also add to your home gym as you progress. For instance, foam rollers and other recovery and mobility tools are some great tools to add as you begin to move into your fitness routine.

I've put together a list of my recommended products on my website as well as links to buy them.

primelifepress.com/rbgear

SCAN HERE

Workout Wear

Now that you have your gym set up and well-kitted out, you need your workout wear. The key is functionality and comfort, you want to wear clothes that are comfortable to move in and do not get in the way of your movements.

Look for items that are breathable and moisture-wicking. Fabric that absorbs sweat will help you cool down and keep a regular body temperature, plus you will feel more comfortable instead of sweaty and clammy.

Your clothing should fit well but not be too tight. You want room to move freely, but you also do not want your shirt flying over your face if you bend down.

For women, a good workout bra should be supportive and comfortable.

You can either work out barefoot or in shoes. Do not work out in socks and this is a slipping hazard. You need shoes that offer a good grip and stability.

Consider Storage

It is easy for small bits and pieces to get tossed aside and leave your space cluttered. I have listed storage boxes as a must-have basic piece of gym equipment as you do need to find solutions to storing your bands, mats, skipping ropes, and any other pieces of gym-associated items.

You could also use shelves or hooks to hang items off.

Choosing the Right Resistance Bands

Different muscle groups and different exercises will require resistance bands in a variety of different strengths to suit the muscle groups being worked. You will need three types of bands which offer light, medium, and heavy resistance. This will support most of your requirements and help build progressive overload while training.

Progressive overload is when you add more intensity to a movement to make it more difficult. You can do this by adding more resistance, more reps, more weight, or more intensity to your exercises. This places additional stress on your muscles, which forces them to adapt and become stronger (Fischer, 2022).

In this case, progressive overload can be achieved by making the resistance harder and using a stronger band.

The light to medium bands can be used for low-impact movements and to work for the smaller muscle groups. These are usually used for upper-body workouts, whereas the heavier bands are more suitable for lower-body work.

Resistance bands are color-coded based on their strength, with the lighter bands usually a lighter color such as yellow and the stronger bands being darker such as blue and black.

There are numerous types of resistance bands, ranging from bands with handles to simple therapy bands. Here are some of your options:

- Latex or fabric loop bands are the most common and popular resistance bands used. They are mini-looped bands that can be used for a variety of different exercises.
- Therapy bands are thinner with less resistance and are used for stretching and mobility work.
- Ankle resistance bands are designed solely for leg movements such as side steps or leg lifts.

- Figure eight bands are similar to loop bands but have a handle.
- Tube bands have handles and are commonly used to perform exercises that you would do with a dumbbell.
- Power resistance bands are longer bands that are commonly used for body weight assistance such as pull-ups (Finlay, 2023).

My advice is to buy a variety of different resistance bands if your budget allows, and do not skimp when it comes to quality. The last thing you want is for your band to get sticky and snap mid-exercise.

Latex versus fabric is up to personal preference, but I find that fabric bands ride up less often during exercise and are very effective for lower-body workouts. Rubber bands offer more stretch and I prefer them for more explosive movements, joint stability exercises, and upper body work.

A simple set of bands is all you need to get a really good workout, but there are accessories available that you can purchase to add to your equipment. Handles, ankle cuffs, and door handles are additional items you could look into purchasing to add to your gym.

Safety Considerations

Start Where You Are

You have done your medical check and your doctor has given you the green light to begin exercising. I understand that you are excited, motivated, and eager to begin your health and fitness journey and want to get started right away and make up for all the missed opportunities.

Instead of diving right into a five-day-a-week workout program, I want to suggest that ease into it slowly. Not only will this set you up for success mentally as we discussed earlier but also physically.

Your body needs to be comfortable with the new movements and stimulus you are putting on it, which can lead to some stiffness and muscle pain. The rest will help you recover and get stronger.

So not only do we avoid injury, but we also avoid potential burnout and boredom.

Once you get more comfortable with the exercise and have familiarized yourself with the movements, do not overdo it. Do not push past more than what feels comfortable for you.

Stick to your program and adjust the exercises if need be depending on any injuries, stiffness, or a general feeling of well-being on that day. Use your workout notes; if you feel particularly sore overall or in one spot, look over your notes. It could be an exercise you were doing, you could have not eaten properly that day or slept well.

Be Aware of Your Surroundings

Before you begin exercising, take a moment to observe your workout area and make sure it is safe. If you are using a chair, secure it and make sure it is stable and will not slide on the flooring. Put any equipment that you are not using away from your workout space.

It is also a good idea to check your bands for general wear and tear before using them in your session. You do not want them to snap mid-exercise.

Stay Hydrated

Sip on water throughout your workout to keep you hydrated. Lack of hydration can result in cramping, headaches, nausea, dizziness, and low blood pressure (Fancy, 2020).

Water keeps your joints lubricated, helps you recover, and improves performance.

Warm Up and Cool Down

An effective warm-up with prepare your muscles for the tasks you are asking them to do, essentially it tells them to get ready for exercise.

There are several reasons why a warm-up and cool-down are important. Let's begin with the warm-up. A warm-up raises your core temperature and gets the blood pumping around the body, it allows your body to gently ease into the movements it is about to perform. Her heart rate slowly rises and the pressure for it to perform is raised gradually and safely. A warm-up lessens the chance of injury, plus it helps recovery by reducing the likelihood of getting stiff or sore afterward.

A warm-up also lets you mentally prepare for the workout.

A cool-down lets your body return to its original state before working out, this is done gently so that you transition smoothly between the two. You could get dizzy or feel a drop in your blood pressure should you just abruptly stop exercising, as a good cool down helps you to regulate your blood flow and slow your heart rate down.

Cool-downs also help initiate recovery and can help reduce muscle soreness and stiffness after exercise. A good cool-down also helps prevent injury and allows you to mentally relax and return to everyday activities (Frey, 2015).

Chapter 3: Warm-Up and Cool-Down

We touched briefly on the importance of warm-ups and cool-downs from a safety perspective in the previous chapters. We will delve into more depth and provide a list of warm-up and cool-down movements you can use to prepare for your workouts.

Warm-Up

According to Bucci (2020), warm-ups have the following benefits:

- Increase the blood and oxygen that is sent to the joints and muscles.
- Increase the dilation of our blood vessels, so blood can be circulated easily.
- Increase the elasticity of our muscles.
- Increase the temperature of our muscles.
- Activate our sweat glands so we do not overheat.
- Reduce the risk of injury.
- Release hormones that convert carbohydrates and fatty acids into energy (Bucci, 2020).

The following movements should be done with intention and control—there is no need to rush any of the following movements.

A good warm-up begins with a cardio-based routine to get the blood flowing, then a ballistic warm-up, which is a combination of slow, gentle, and rhythmic movements. You can choose a cardio piece that you feel comfortable with and then continue by selecting the exercises that are most appropriate for the work you have programmed to do.

If you are focusing on your upper body, then your warm-up should have an upper body focus and vice versa. You could also do a full-body warm-up as well. Have fun and experiment with your warm-up routines, there are no hard and fast rules.

Cardio-Based Warm Up Exercises

MARCHING

View a demo of this exercise by scanning the QR code or going to: primelifepress.com/rbwu1

1. Begin by standing up tall with your shoulder blades back and down. Your arms should be at your side and your feet placed underneath your hips.
2. Bending at the knee, raise your left leg as high as it feels comfortable while swinging your right arm in a marching motion.
3. Return your leg to the ground and your arm back to your side.
4. Repeat on the other side.
5. Continue this marching motion for your allocated amount of time.
6. Thirty seconds to a minute is a good place to start.

SCAN FOR VIDEO

WALKING/JUMPING JACKS

View a demo of this exercise by scanning the QR code or going to: primelifepress.com/rbwu2

1. Begin by standing up tall with your shoulder blades back and down. Your arms should be at your side and your feet placed underneath your hips.
2. Take a lateral step with your left leg out to your left side.
3. While you are taking your step, swing both arms out to your sides and extend them upwards so that they meet overhead.
4. Lower your arms back to the starting position while returning your left leg to the middle.
5. Repeat on the other side.
6. If you are doing jumping jacks, jump both feet out laterally at the same time while extending your arms overhead. Finish by jumping them back to the center and lowering your arms.
7. Continue your walking/jumping jacks for your allocated amount of time.
8. Thirty seconds to a minute is a good place to start.

SCAN FOR VIDEO

KNEES TO ELBOW MARCHING

View a demo of this exercise by scanning the QR code or going to: primelifepress.com/rbwu3

1. Begin by standing up tall with your shoulder blades back and down. Your arms should be at your side and your feet placed underneath your hips.
2. Bending at the knee, raise your left leg as high as it feels comfortable.
3. Return your leg to the ground.
4. Repeat on the other side.
5. Continue this marching motion for 10 repetitions.
6. Now incorporate your arms.
7. As you raise your leg, bring your opposite elbow to meet your opposite knee.
8. Return to the starting position and repeat on the other side.
9. Continue for your allocated amount of time.

SCAN FOR VIDEO

SHADOW BOXING

View a demo of this exercise by scanning the QR code or going to: primelifepress.com/rbwu4

1. Begin by standing up tall with your shoulder blades back and down. Your arms should be at your side and your feet placed underneath your hips.
2. Bring both of your hands in close to your chest, creating fists.
3. Extend your right fist forward and straighten your arm in a punching motion.
4. Return it to your chest while extending your left fist forward in a punching motion.
5. Continue for your allocated amount of time.

SCAN FOR VIDEO

LATERAL SIDE STEPS

View a demo of this exercise by scanning the QR code or going to: primelifepress.com/rbwu5

1. Begin by standing up tall with your shoulder blades back and down. Your arms should be at your side and your feet placed underneath your hips.
2. Bring your hands up to the center of your chest.
3. Bend your knees slightly.
4. Take a lateral step with your left leg out to your left side.
5. Bring your right leg to meet your left leg so that both feet are together.
6. Take a lateral step with your right leg out to your right side.
7. Bring your left leg to meet your right leg so that both feet are together.
8. Continue for your allocated amount of time.
9. Thirty seconds is a good place to start.

SHUFFLE STEPS

View a demo of this exercise by scanning the QR code or going to: primelifepress.com/rbwu6

1. Begin by standing up tall with your shoulder blades back and down. Your arms should be at your side and your feet placed underneath your hips.
2. Take a step forward with your right leg and bring your left leg to meet it.
3. Take another step forward with your right leg and bring your left leg to meet it.
4. Take a step backward with your left leg, and bring your right leg back to meet it.
5. Take another step backward with your left leg, and bring your right leg back to meet it.
6. Repeat on the same leg for your allocated amount of time.
7. Fifteen seconds is a good place to start.
8. Repeat with the other foot.

SCAN FOR VIDEO

BOX STEPS

View a demo of this exercise by scanning the QR code or going to: primelifepress.com/rbwu7

1. Begin by standing up tall with your shoulder blades back and down. Your arms should be at your side and your feet placed underneath your hips.
2. Leading with your right leg, take a lateral step to your right.
3. Take a step forward with your right leg.
4. Switch to your left leg and take a lateral step to your left.
5. Take a step backward with your left leg.
6. Repeat the sequence for your allocated amount of time.

SCAN FOR VIDEO

HEEL DIGS

View a demo of this exercise by scanning the QR code or going to: primelifepress.com/rbwu8

1. Begin by standing up tall with your shoulder blades back and down. Your arms should be at your side and your feet placed underneath your hips.
2. Extend your left leg out straight in front of you and tap your heel to the ground.
3. Return to your starting position.
4. Extend your right leg out straight in front of you and tap your heel to the ground.
5. Return to your starting position.
6. Repeat the sequence for your allocated amount of time.

TOE TAPS AND PRESS

View a demo of this exercise by scanning the QR code or going to: primelifepress.com/rbwu10

1. Begin by standing up tall with your shoulder blades back and down. Your arms should be raised at your chest and your feet placed underneath your hips.
2. Extend your left leg out straight out behind you and tap your toes to the ground.
3. As you do so, push your arms forward and extend them in front of your chest.
4. Return to your starting position.
5. Extend your right leg out straight out behind you and tap your toes to the ground.
6. As you do so, push your arms forward and extend them in front of your chest.
7. Return to your starting position.
8. Repeat the sequence for your allocated amount of time.

BUTT KICKS

View a demo of this exercise by scanning the QR code or going to: primelifepress.com/rbwu11

1. Begin by standing up tall with your shoulder blades back and down. Your arms should be at your side and your feet placed underneath your hips.
2. Bend your right leg towards your buttocks and bend as far back as comfortable, aim to touch the back of your leg with your heel.
3. Return to starting position.
4. Bend your left leg towards your buttocks and bend as far back as comfortable, aim to touch the back of your leg with your heel.
5. Return to starting position.
6. Repeat, alternating each leg, for your allocated amount of time.

Mobilty-Based Warm Up Exercises

HEAD ROLLS

View a demo of this exercise by scanning the QR code or going to: primelifepress.com/rbwu12

1. Begin by standing or sitting up tall in a chair with your shoulders down and back.
2. Tuck your chin down towards your chest.
3. Gently roll your head to the left, passing your shoulder, extending backward, and coming past your right should to return to the starting position.
4. Repeat the head rolls for the required amount of repetitions, 10 - 15 is the average rep range.
5. Repeat in the other direction.

SCAN FOR VIDEO

NECK ROTATIONS

View a demo of this exercise by scanning the QR code or going to: primelifepress.com/rbwu13

1. Begin by standing or sitting up tall in a chair with your shoulders down and back.
2. Keeping your torso facing forward and only moving your head, gently turn to look over your right shoulder.
3. Return to center.
4. Keeping your torso facing forward and only moving your head, gently turn to look over your left shoulder.
5. Repeat the neck rotations for the required amount of repetitions, 10-16 is the average rep range.

SCAN FOR VIDEO

NECK LATERAL FLEXION

View a demo of this exercise by scanning the QR code or going to: primelifepress.com/rbwu14

1. Begin by standing or sitting up tall in a chair with your shoulders down and back.
2. Keeping your torso facing forward, gently bend your right ear towards your right shoulder.
3. Return to center.
4. Keeping your torso facing forward, gently bend your left ear towards your left shoulder.
5. Repeat the neck lateral flexion for the required amount of repetitions, 10-16 is the average rep range.

SCAN FOR VIDEO

WRIST ROTATIONS

View a demo of this exercise by scanning the QR code or going to: primelifepress.com/rbwu15

1. Begin by raising your arms in front of you and clenching your hands into a fist.
2. Moving from your wrists, rotate your hands inwards in a circular motion.
3. Repeat for the required amount of reps, 10 is the average rep range.
4. Repeat the wrist rotations by rotating your hand outwards.

SCAN FOR VIDEO

FOREARM CIRCLES

View a demo of this exercise by scanning the QR code or going to: primelifepress.com/rbwu16

1. Begin by tucking your elbows into the side of your body and raising your forearms so that they are parallel to the floor with your palms facing forward.
2. Moving from your elbows, slowly rotate your forearms forward in circles.
3. Repeat for the required amount of reps, 10 is the average rep range.
4. Repeat the forearm circles in opposite directions.

SCAN FOR VIDEO

ARM CIRCLES

View a demo of this exercise by scanning the QR code or going to: primelifepress.com/rbwu17

1. Begin by standing tall with your shoulders down and back and your feet under your hips.
2. Straighten your arms out to your side and, moving from your shoulders, rotate them in wide circles forward.
3. Repeat for the required amount of repetitions, 10-15 is the average rep range.
4. Repeat your arms circles in the other direction.

SCAN FOR VIDEO

SHOULDER ROLLS

View a demo of this exercise by scanning the QR code or going to: primelifepress.com/rbwu18

1. Begin by standing or sitting up tall in a chair with your shoulders down and back.
2. Shrug your shoulders up to your ears.
3. Roll them backward and down, squeezing your shoulder blades together.
4. Repeat this movement for the required amount of repetitions, 10–12 repetitions is an average rep range.

T-ARM ROTATION

View a demo of this exercise by scanning the QR code or going to: primelifepress.com/rbwu19

1. Begin by standing up tall with your shoulders back and down and your feet placed under your hips.
2. Raise both your arms to the side in line with your shoulders with your palms facing upwards.
3. Keeping your shoulder blades engaged, slowly rotate your palms down towards the floor and all the way around until they are facing behind you.
4. Reverse the motions and rotate them back towards the ceiling.
5. Repeat for the required amount of repetition, 8–10 is the average rep range.

THORACIC ROTATION

View a demo of this exercise by scanning the QR code or going to: primelifepress.com/rbwu20

1. Begin by standing tall with your shoulders back and down and your feet placed under your hips.
2. Cross your arms over your chest.
3. Leading with your arms, rotate just your upper body towards the right until you feel a stretch in your upper back.
4. Hold for three seconds and rotate to the other side.
5. Repeat for the set amount of repetitions, five on each side is the average rep range.

SCAN FOR VIDEO

BOW AND BENDS

View a demo of this exercise by scanning the QR code or going to: primelifepress.com/rbwu21

1. Begin by standing tall with your shoulders back and down and your feet placed under your hips.
2. Fold forward gently, hinging from your hips, and relax your upper body.
3. Let your arms and upper body hang freely.
4. Slowly roll back up, vertebrae by vertebrae, until you are standing tall.
5. Repeat for five repetitions.

SCAN FOR VIDEO

HIP ROTATIONS

View a demo of this exercise by scanning the QR code or going to: primelifepress.com/rbwu22

1. Begin by standing tall with your shoulders back and down and your feet placed under your hips. If you require a chair for balance, stand to the side of it.
2. Raise your left knee as high as comfortable and rotate it outwards to the left.
3. Your leg should still be bent with the knee facing towards the left and the sole of your foot in line with your calf.
4. Rotate it back to the center.
5. Place your foot on the floor.
6. Swap sides.
7. Repeat and alternate each leg for five repetitions each leg.

SCAN FOR VIDEO

LEG SWINGS

View a demo of this exercise by scanning the QR code or going to: primelifepress.com/rbwu23

1. Begin by standing tall next to your chair with your shoulders back and down and your feet placed under your hips. Place your hand on the back of the chair for balance.
2. Keeping your right leg straight, swing it in front of you as high as you feel comfortable.
3. Let it return and swing it backward. Keep your upper body as still as possible, swinging only from the hip.
4. Swing your leg back and forth for 20 repetitions.
5. Swap legs.

ANKLE CIRCLES

View a demo of this exercise by scanning the QR code or going to: primelifepress.com/rbwu24

1. Begin by sitting up tall in your chair with your shoulders down and back.
2. Your feet should be placed under your knees.
3. Lift your left leg off the floor and point your toes.
4. Rotate your ankle outwards for 10 repetitions.
5. Repeat in the opposite direction.
6. Lift your right leg off the floor and point your toes.
7. Rotate your ankle outwards for 10 repetitions.
8. Repeat in the opposite direction.

SCAN FOR VIDEO

ANKLE FLEXION

View a demo of this exercise by scanning the QR code or going to: primelifepress.com/rbwu25

1. Begin by sitting up tall in your chair with your shoulders down and back.
2. Your feet should be placed under your knees.
3. Lift your left leg off the floor.
4. Point your toe forward, then point your toes back towards your body.
5. You should feel a stretch in your calf. Repeat for 10 repetitions.
6. Lift your right leg off the floor.
7. Point your toe forward, then point your toes back towards your body.
8. You should feel a stretch in your calf. Repeat for 10 repetitions.

Cool-Downs

Cooling down allows your body to slowly return to its normal state, where the heart rate slows down, and your muscles begin to relax post-workout.

A basic cool-down consists of a few minutes of slow cardio followed by some stretching or rehab/prehab exercises.

You can incorporate one of the cardio warm-up exercises listed previously in the chapter and perform it at a more relaxed pace as a cool-down. Then add one or two of the stretches and movements below, depending on what exercises you have done for the day.

SCAN FOR VIDEO

CAT/COW STRETCH

View a demo of this exercise by scanning the QR code or going to: primelifepress.com/rbcd1

1. Begin on the floor on all fours. Your hands should be placed underneath your shoulders and your knees underneath your hips.
2. Look upwards towards the ceiling, only moving your neck.
3. Drop your belly towards the ground while tilting your pelvis upwards.
4. Flex your neck downwards, so you are looking towards your belly.
5. Tuck your pelvis downwards and pull your navel to your spine.
6. Arch back and forth like this for five repetitions.

SCAN FOR VIDEO

FORWARD BEND

View a demo of this exercise by scanning the QR code or going to: primelifepress.com/rbcd2

1. Begin by standing tall with your shoulders back and down and your feet placed under your hips.
2. Fold forward gently, hinging from your hips, and reach for your toes.
3. Roll slowly back up, extending your arms over your head and actively reaching for the ceiling.
4. Repeat for five repetitions.

SCAN FOR VIDEO

HAMSTRING STRETCH

View a demo of this exercise by scanning the QR code or going to: primelifepress.com/rbcd3

1. Begin by standing tall with your shoulders back and down and your feet placed under your hips. You can use a chair to help keep you balanced.
2. Keeping your leg straight, place one foot in front of you and keep both heels on the ground.
3. Keep the toes of your back leg facing forward and soften your knee.
4. Keep your back straight and your hips facing forward, and you lean towards your front leg.
5. You should feel a stretch in the back of your leg.
6. Hold for the set time.
7. Swap legs.

SCAN FOR VIDEO

QUADRUPED STRETCH

View a demo of this exercise by scanning the QR code or going to: primelifepress.com/rbcd4

1. Begin by standing tall with your shoulders back and down and your feet placed under your hips. You can use a chair to help keep you balanced.
2. Holding onto your foot, bring your left leg up and behind you, pulling your heel to your glutes.
3. Keep your back straight and upright, and keep your knees together.
4. Hold for a set amount of time.
5. Swap legs.

SCAN FOR VIDEO

CALF STRETCH

View a demo of this exercise by scanning the QR code or going to: primelifepress.com/rbcd5

1. Begin by standing tall with your shoulders back and down and your feet placed under your hips. Hold onto the back of a chair for balance.
2. Keep your toes facing forward and take a step back with your right leg.
3. Keep your heels on the ground and gently bring your front knee toward the chair.
4. Lean gently into the stretch.
5. Hold for a set amount of time.
6. Swap legs.

SCAN FOR VIDEO

ABDUCTOR STRETCH

View a demo of this exercise by scanning the QR code or going to: primelifepress.com/rbcd6

1. Begin by standing tall with your shoulders back and down and your feet placed under your hips.
2. Step your right leg out to the side, keeping both feet with their toes pointing forward or slightly out to the side.
3. Gently bend your right leg and shift your weight onto it, keeping your left leg straight as you lean.
4. Keep your left foot planted firmly on the ground.
5. You should feel a stretch in your inner thigh.
6. Hold for a short amount of time.
7. Swap legs.

SCAN FOR

VIDEO

SEATED HIP FLEXION STRETCH

View a demo of this exercise by scanning the QR code or going to: primelifepress.com/rbcd7

1. Begin by sitting upright in your chair with your shoulders down and back.
2. Keep your feet underneath your knees.
3. Bring your right knee up towards your chest and pull it as close as comfortable to your chest, keeping your back straight.
4. Hold for the set amount of time and release.
5. Swap legs.

SCAN FOR VIDEO

SEATED HIP LATERAL ROTATION STRETCH

View a demo of this exercise by scanning the QR code or going to: primelifepress.com/rbcd8

1. Begin by sitting upright towards the front of your chair, with your shoulders down and back.
2. Keep your feet underneath your knees.
3. Cross your right leg over your left and rest your ankle on the top of your knee.
4. Place your hands on the shins of your bent leg and slowly lean forward.
5. Hold for a set amount of time and release.
6. Swap legs.

SCAN FOR VIDEO

LUMBAR SIDE STRETCH

View a demo of this exercise by scanning the QR code or going to: primelifepress.com/rbcd9

1. Begin by sitting upright in your chair with your shoulders down and back.
2. Keep your feet underneath your knees.
3. Let your left arm hang straight at your side and place your right hand behind your head.
4. Gently lean down towards your left, letting your left arm slide straight downward. You should feel a stretch on the opposite side.
5. Hold for the set amount of time and release.
6. Swap sides.

SCAN FOR VIDEO

LOWER BACK STRETCH

View a demo of this exercise by scanning the QR code or going to: primelifepress.com/rbcd10

1. Begin by standing up tall with your shoulders down and back.
2. Place your hands on the small of your back.
3. Gently lean backward into your hands.
4. Hold for the set amount of time and release.

SCAN FOR VIDEO

OVERHEAD STRETCH

View a demo of this exercise by scanning the QR code or going to: primelifepress.com/rbcd11

1. Begin by standing up tall with your shoulders down and back.
2. Lace your fingers together and bring them up overhead.
3. Turn your palms to face the ceiling.
4. Push up as far as you can. You should feel a stretch in your sides and your shoulders.
5. Hold for a set amount of time and release.

SCAN FOR

VIDEO

BICEP AND SHOULDER STRETCH

View a demo of this exercise by scanning the QR code or going to: primelifepress.com/rbcd12

1. Begin by standing up tall with your shoulders down and back.
2. Place your right arm straight across your body.
3. Use your other hand to hug your right arm close to your chest.
4. Hold for the set amount of time and release.
5. Swap sides.

SCAN FOR VIDEO

TRICEPS STRETCH

View a demo of this exercise by scanning the QR code or going to: primelifepress.com/rbcd13

1. Begin by standing up tall with your shoulders down and back.

2. Place your right palm behind your head, in between your shoulder blades.

SCAN FOR
VIDEO

CHEST OPENER

View a demo of this exercise by scanning the QR code or going to: primelifepress.com/rbcd14

1. Begin by standing up tall with your shoulders down and back.
2. Raise your arms in front of you so that they are parallel to the floor.
3. Slowly bring your arms out to the side and pull as far back as you feel comfortable.
4. Squeeze your shoulder blades together but ensure that you are maintaining a straight back and upright posture.
5. Hold for the set amount of time and release.

All of these exercises can be done seated as well or with the use of a chair for support and balance. Feel free to experiment with the warm-ups and cool-downs, the cool-down stretches can also be done as a relaxing movement and stretching piece on your days off from exercise.

Chapter 4: Strengthening Muscles for Better Posture and Mobility

The Importance of Muscle Strength

We need to stay strong and active during our older years, which means it is essential for us to focus on maintaining or building muscle mass. We have touched briefly on why muscle mass is important, and now we will look a little closer as to why.

The opposite of strong is frail, and we do not want to go into old age frail. We do not want to be physically weak, nor do we want to be so mentally. Strengthening our muscles can also result in strengthening our minds, feeling strong physically can also promote mental and emotional health.

Strength training activities such as resistance band training can help in the following areas:

- build strength
- maintain bone density
- reduce your risks of falls

- improve balance and coordination
- improve mobility
- maintain independence (Seguin et al., 2003)

The exercises we have put together here require little time and equipment but create great rewards.

Some of these perks are a reduction in the symptoms of certain diseases and ailments such as arthritis, diabetes, osteoporosis, heart disease, obesity, and a reduction in back pain.

Resistance training can also help you fall asleep easier and sleep sounder. Symptoms of depression and anxiety may decrease, and you may feel a rise in self-confidence and self-esteem.

We are going to do a long-term experiment now. This will give you an indication of your progress and why we want to be strength training well into our older years.

The following log will track how fit and strong you are over the space of a year (I have confidence that you will be able to reach this milestone easily). When you are done reading this book, fill out the log by filling in your scores and adding them up. Make a note of your current fitness levels. You will then revisit it over the space of three, six, and twelve months to determine if there has been any change.

How Fit and Strong Are You Now?

Rarely (1 point) Sometimes (2 points) Usually (3 points) Always (4 points)

Daily Activities	Start	3 Months	6 Months	9 Months	12 Months
It is easy for me to walk up and down flights of stairs.					
I can take out the trash easily.					
I can vacuum, dust, and do other housework unaided.					
I can easily lift a gallon of milk.					

I have no trouble bending down to get something off the floor or reaching up to higher shelves.					
I find it easy to do outdoor gardening work such as raking or mowing the lawn.					
Mood, Energy Levels, and Mental Health	Start	3 Months	6 Months	9 Months	12 Months
I am as active as other people my age.					
I feel healthy.					

I feel strong.					
I feel energetic.					
I feel independent.					
I live an active life.					
I feel younger than my age.					
Total					

Evaluate your results:

15—29 points: Fitness levels are considered low. A lot of room to improve mobility, the ability to complete daily tasks, as well as mental health and mood.

30—39 points: Low-to-moderate fitness level, with room for improvement in most areas.

40—49 points: Moderate fitness level, with room for improvement in some of the above areas.

50+ points: Advanced fitness level; strength training will improve and maintain fitness.

You can use this information to plan your goals and work on areas of your life that have been neglected and need some work.

Age and Posture Change

Do you find that you hold yourself differently when sitting or standing up? Small postural changes are a common symptom of aging, but more major changes, such as hyperkyphosis, may also occur. Kyphosis is characterized as a hunchback and affects the thoracic spine, which is situated between the lower back and neck.

If you do notice changes in your posture, whether they are minor or major, it is best that you talk to your doctor. They can evaluate your need for intervention as there can be possible issues, in addition to discomfort that may occur; such as breathing problems, balance issues, and problems with completing certain day-to-day tasks.

When we are, there are three main "areas" that are affected. There are your muscles, the vertebrae (this is the column of bones that run along your spine), and the disks in your back. These disks cushion your vertebrae.

As we get older, we see a loss of bone density, which is known as osteoporosis if severe, and osteopenia if milder. These ailments cause the vertebrae to lose calcium, become less dense, and shrink. As your bones become weaker, they shrink and your posture may change.

Muscle loss occurs as we age, which reduces the support we have around our bones and joints. As we lose the support around our spine, we find that our torso no longer stays as upright as before, resulting in a hunched back.

Finally, the disks in our back are prone to shrinkage as the years go by. These are responsible for providing cushioning between our vertebrae, and as they get smaller the bones get closer and our movement patterns begin to change.

As I have continually stressed throughout this book—these changes do not have to happen. We can easily alter our path by exercising for a few hours a week. By keeping our chest, back, shoulder, and neck muscles strong, we can keep our body aligned and moving correctly. Our range of motion, mobility, flexibility, and movement patterns will all benefit (Cristol, 2021).

Besides exercising, what else can you do to improve your posture?

The first thing you can do is to be mindful of the way that you are holding and moving your body. This is especially important when you begin to exercise. We always want to build the correct movement patterns, and each repetition we do when we are exercising can either set us back or move us forward. It should never be so difficult to do a repetition that your form falters.

Breathe deeply and consciously as often as you remember, this too makes you more mindful of your body creates physical awareness, and helps move your body back into good positions.

Modify your environment so that it makes it easy for you to practice standing up or sitting up straight. Simple changes to your desk, chair, and computer can work wonders and bring great changes to the way you position yourself while working and when you are not. Change the height of your computer, use a footstool, or invest in a standing desk.

Take a moment to relax your muscles, especially those in your neck and shoulders. Relax your abdomen and keep your feet planted firmly on the ground and underneath your hips. Your knees should be relaxed and your head in line with your spine.

When sitting, check in with yourself and see if you are slouching or rounding your shoulders.

The Role of Resistance Bands in Improving Posture

Resistance bands can work both your bigger muscles and the smaller muscles, which are known as stabilizers. The stabilizing muscles support our joints and larger muscles. Having strong stabilizer muscles can reduce our chances of injury.

By creating strength in our shoulders, upper and lower back, core muscles as well as neck we can maintain the strength that we need to keep our posture good.

Because resistance band movements often require concentration and control, we can develop a greater sense of body awareness and mindfulness of movement—important skills to have when focusing on improving our posture.

Chapter 5: Resistance Band Exercises

This chapter should be considered your exercise library. I have collected numerous resistance band movements and compiled them into the following sections:

- upper body
- lower body
- full body

Most of these exercises can also be performed seated or with support from a chair. When selecting the right resistance band for the exercise, consider choosing a band that allows you to reach moderate to maximum muscle fatigue between 20–30 reps. If you can do 20 repetitions without too much of an effort, then the band is too easy for you, but if you can only do 2–4 it is too light.

Some key points to remember when performing your movements:

- Avoid holding your breath during movements.
- Breathe out during the hardest part of the movement.

- Perform your movements in a slow and controlled manner.
- Use the full range of motion around each joint and muscle that is worked.

EXERCISE 1
BAND PULL APARTS

SCAN FOR VIDEO

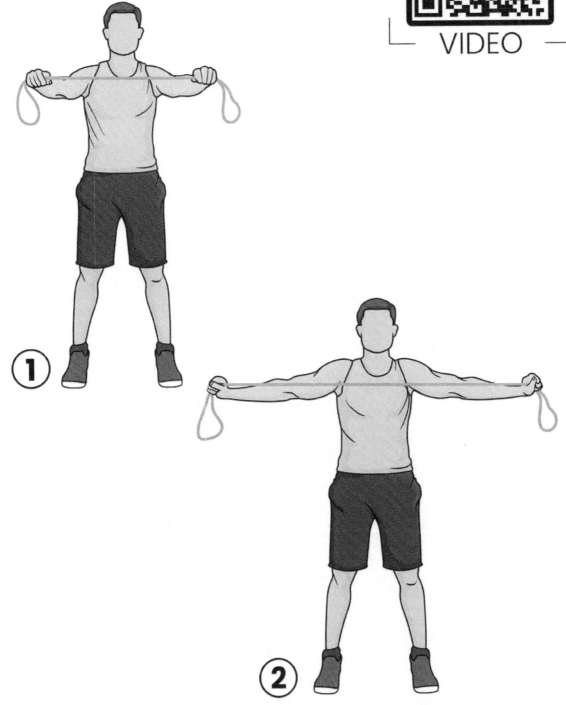

① ②

BAND PULL APARTS

View a demo of this exercise by scanning the QR code or going to: primelifepress.com/rbub1

1. Begin by standing up tall with your shoulders back and down. Your feet should be underneath your hips.
2. Hold the end of the resistance band in each hand.
3. Lift your arms out straight in front of you until they are shoulder height with your palms facing downward. Your hands should be about six inches apart and the band should have slight tension but should not be too taut.
4. Pull the band out to your sides, extending your arms wide, creating a T position.
5. Kelly your hands in line with each other at the same height.
6. When your arms are fully extended, hold the position for two seconds.
7. Return to center.
8. Repeat for the recommended amount of reps. The average is 10 repetitions.

EXERCISE 2
BOW & ARROW

SCAN FOR

VIDEO

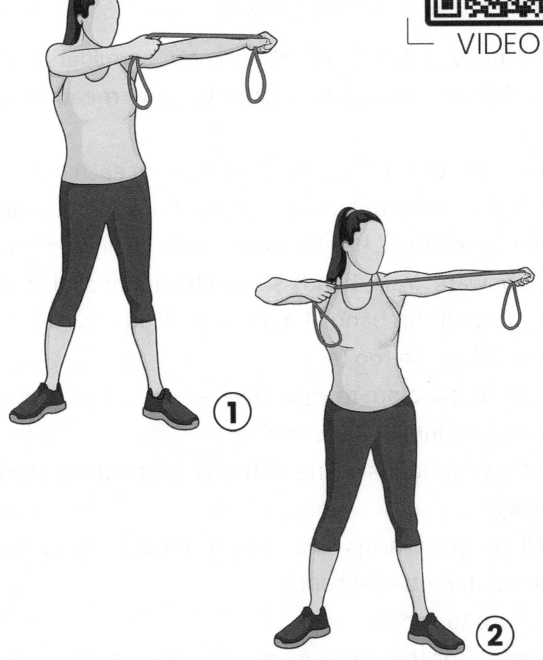

BOW AND ARROW

View a demo of this exercise by scanning the QR code or going to: primelifepress.com/rbub2

1. Begin by standing up tall with your shoulders back and down. Your feet should be underneath your hips and your core engaged.
2. Hold the end of the resistance band in each hand.
3. Raise both of your hands to chest level.
4. Find your starting position by extending your left arm to your left side and keeping your right arm in line with the middle of your chest.
5. Adjust the tension of your band so that there is light tension on the band.
6. Pull your right hand away from your left arm as if you are drawing back an arrow from a bow.
7. Your elbows should be elevated and pointed outwards.
8. Return to the starting position.
9. Repeat for the recommended amount of reps on one side and then swap. The average is 10—12 repetitions per side.

EXERCISE 3
LATERAL RAISE

SCAN FOR VIDEO

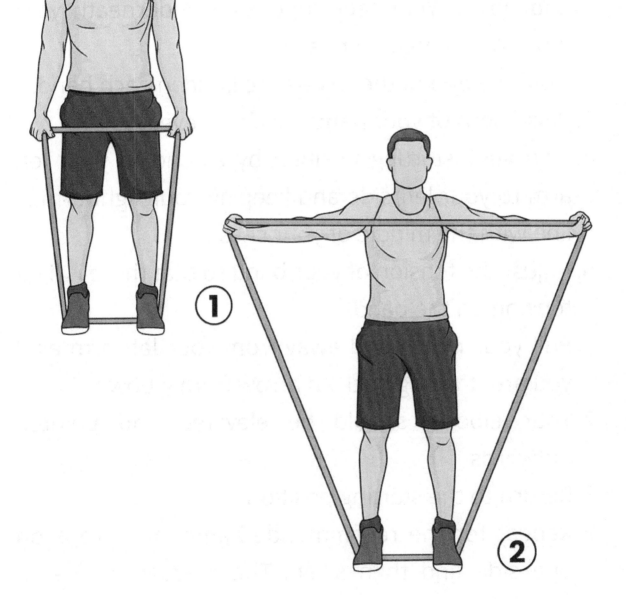

① ②

LATERAL RAISE

View a demo of this exercise by scanning the QR code or going to: primelifepress.com/rbub3

1. Begin by standing up tall with your shoulders back and down. Your feet should be placed underneath your hips.
2. Holding the end of the resistance band in each hand, loop it under both your feet.
3. Raise your arms to your side until they are in line with your shoulder blades.
4. Return to the starting position.
5. Repeat for the recommended amount of reps. The average is 10–15 repetitions.

STAGGERED STANCE ROW

SCAN FOR

VIDEO

① ②

STAGGERED STANCE ROW

View a demo of this exercise by scanning the QR code or going to: primelifepress.com/rbub4

1. Begin by standing up tall with your shoulders back and down.
2. Place your left foot in front of your right so that you are in a staggered stance. Widen your stance slightly if you feel off balance.
3. Holding the end of the resistance band in each hand, loop it under your left foot.
4. Bend your left leg slightly, engage your core, and bend forward from your hip while keeping your back straight.
5. Set up your starting position by extending your arms down towards your left foot.
6. Ensure that the band has light tension.
7. Pull your hands towards your torso in a rowing motion. Keep your elbows, arms, and hands in line with your ribcage.
8. Compete the rep by extending your arms to the starting position.
9. Repeat for the recommended amount of reps on one side and then swap feet. The average is 8—12 repetitions per side.

BENT OVER ROW

SCAN FOR

VIDEO

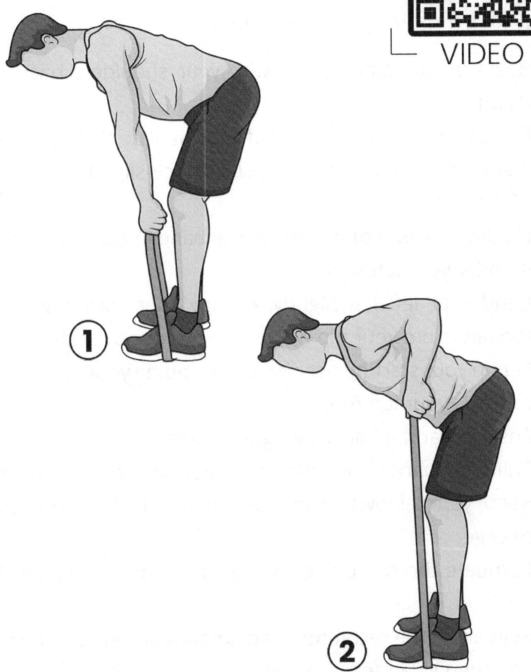

BENT OVER ROW

View a demo of this exercise by scanning the QR code or going to: primelifepress.com/rbub5

1. Begin by standing up tall with your shoulders back and down. Your feet should be underneath your hips.
2. Holding the end of the resistance band in each hand, loop it under both of your feet.
3. Bending forward from your hip, lower your upper body forward so that you are parallel to the floor.
4. Let your arms lower towards your feet.
5. Start the movement by pulling your arms towards your ribcage and allowing your shoulder blades to come together. Your elbows should be pointing up towards the ceiling.
6. Return to the starting point.
7. Repeat for the recommended amount of reps. The average is 10–15 repetitions.

EXERCISE 6
SEATED ROW

SCAN FOR

VIDEO

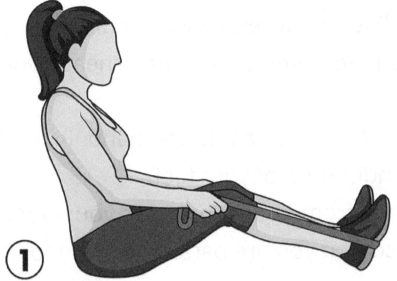

①

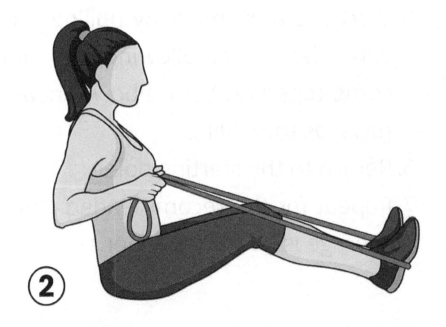

②

SEATED ROW

View a demo of this exercise by scanning the QR code or going to: primelifepress.com/rbub6

1. Begin by sitting on the floor with your legs stretched out in front of you.
2. Loop your resistance band around the soles of your feet and hold each end of the back with your palms facing each other.
3. Bend your knees slightly.
4. Keeping your back straight and your elbows close to your sides, pull the band towards your navel.
5. When your arms reach a 90° angle, squeeze your shoulder blades together and slowly return to the starting position.
6. Repeat for the recommended amount of reps. The average is 10–15 repetitions.

EXERCISE 7
BANDED FRONT RAISE

SCAN FOR VIDEO

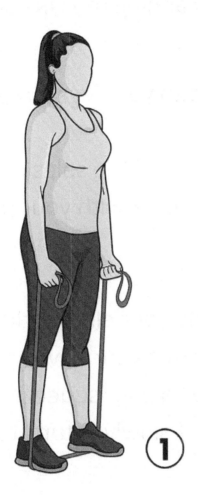
①

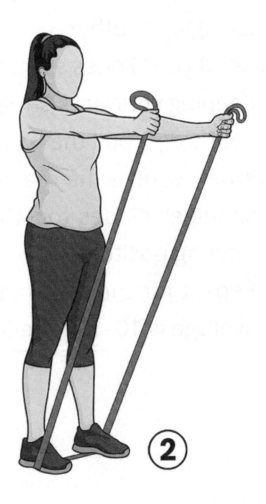
②

BANDED FRONT RAISE

View a demo of this exercise by scanning the QR code or going to: primelifepress.com/rbub7

1. Begin by standing up tall with your shoulders back and down. Your feet should be underneath your hips.
2. Holding the end of the resistance band in each hand, loop it under both of your feet.
3. Pull the band up in front of you, keeping your arms straight.
4. Stop when you reach shoulder height.
5. Return to the starting position.
6. Repeat for the recommended amount of reps. The average is 10–15 repetitions.

EXERCISE 8
CUFF PIVOT

SCAN FOR VIDEO

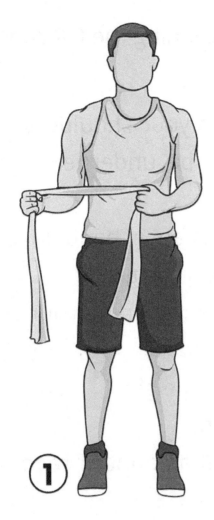

①

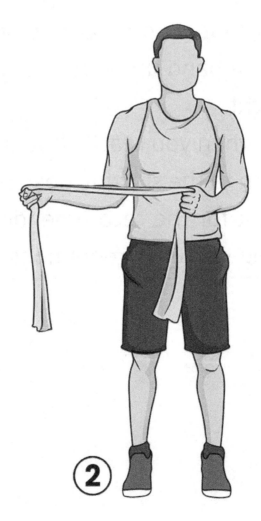

②

CUFF PIVOT

View a demo of this exercise by scanning the QR code or going to: primelifepress.com/rbub8

1. Begin by standing up tall with your shoulders back and down. Engage your core.
2. Hold each end of the resistance band in your hands, just below your chest and in line with the bottom of your ribcage.
3. Bend your elbows and point them outwards.
4. You should be using a short band, but if you do not have one, wrap yours around your hand a few times to create tension.
5. Keep your left hand still and pull your right hand outwards. Keep your elbow fixed to your waist and it rotates from the shoulder.
6. Keep your arm bent, focusing on rotating your arm using your shoulder blades.
7. Return to the starting position and repeat on the same side for the recommended amount of reps. The average is 10–12 reps on one side.

EXERCISE 9
CHEST PRESS

SCAN FOR VIDEO

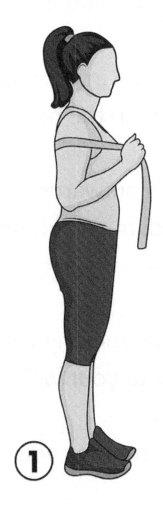
①

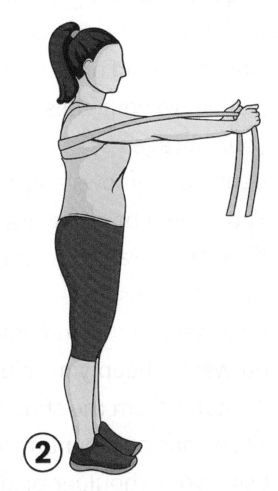
②

CHEST PRESS

View a demo of this exercise by scanning the QR code or going to: primelifepress.com/rbub9

1. Begin by standing up tall with your shoulders back and down. Engage your core.
2. Hold each end of the resistance band in your hands and place the middle section of it behind your upper back. It should be in line with your shoulders.
3. Extend your arms in front of you with the palms facing downward.
4. Return to the starting position.
5. Repeat for the recommended amount of reps. The average is 10–15 repetitions.

SCAPULAR RETRACTION

SCAN FOR VIDEO

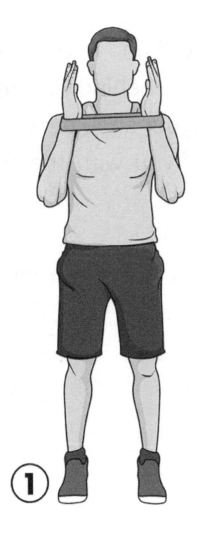

①

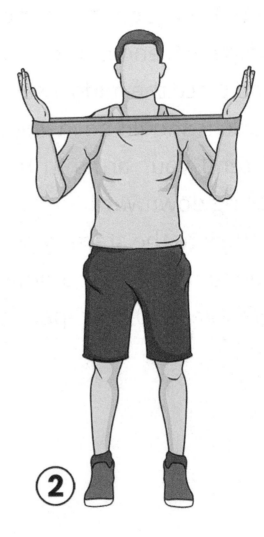

②

SCAPULAR RETRACTION

View a demo of this exercise by scanning the QR code or going to: primelifepress.com/rbub10

1. Begin by standing up tall with your shoulders down and back. Your feet should be underneath your hips.
2. Place your resistance band around your wrists. You may need a shorter band or may have to wrap the band around your wrists a couple of times.
3. With your palms facing forward and your fingers pointing to the ceiling, place your arms at a 90° angle.
4. Slowly rotate your elbows out while squeezing your shoulder blades together. Keep your core tight and your back straight.
5. Pause and squeeze your shoulder blades together for two seconds.
6. Release and return to the starting position.
7. Repeat for the recommended amount of reps. The average is 10–15 repetitions.

EXERCISE 11
OVERHEAD PRESS

SCAN FOR

VIDEO

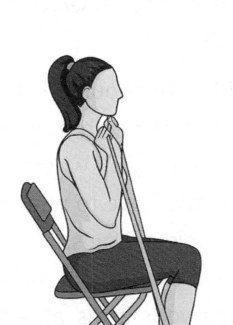

①

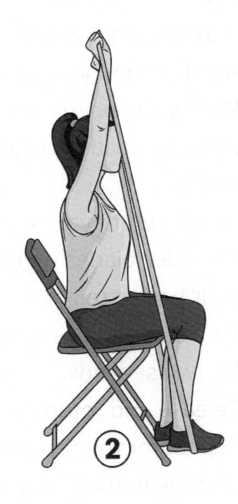

②

OVERHEAD PRESS

View a demo of this exercise by scanning the QR code or going to: primelifepress.com/rbub11

1. Begin by standing up tall with your shoulders down and back. Your feet should be underneath your hips.
2. Loop your resistance band underneath both of your feet and hold each end of the band in one hand at shoulder height.
3. Your palms should be facing forward.
4. Press your arms straight up over your head. Avoid arching backward by keeping your back straight.
5. Lower your arms back down to your collarbone.
6. Repeat for the recommended amount of reps. The average is 8–12 repetitions.

TRICEP EXTENSION

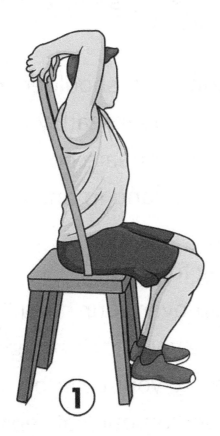

①

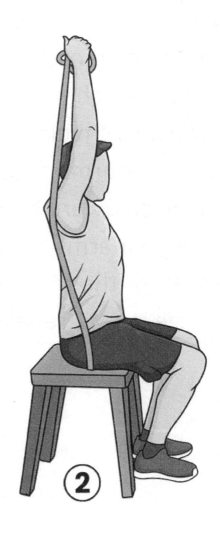

②

OVERHEAD TRICEPS EXTENSION

View a demo of this exercise by scanning the QR code or going to: primelifepress.com/rbub12

1. Begin by standing up tall with your shoulders down and back. Your feet should be close together.
2. Loop your resistance band underneath both of your feet and hold each end of the band behind your head. The band should be running behind your body up along your back.
3. Keep your elbows close to your ears with your palms facing each other and your knuckles touching,
4. This is where you will start.
5. Straighten your elbows without moving your arms, and extend your arms overhead. Keep your elbows close to your ears as you do so, and keep your shoulders down and back and your core engaged.
6. Pause at the top for a second and lower the band behind you.
7. Repeat for the recommended amount of reps. The average is 15–20 repetitions.

OVERHEAD PULL APART

SCAN FOR VIDEO

① ②

OVERHEAD PULL APART

View a demo of this exercise by scanning the QR code or going to: primelifepress.com/rbub13

1. Begin by standing up tall with your shoulders down and back. Your feet should be about shoulder-width apart.
2. Hold the ends of the resistance band in each hand and put your arms overhead, directly above you.
3. As you bring the band down behind your back, pull it apart and stretch it across your shoulders as your hands fully extend to either side.
4. Hold for a second before slowly returning to the starting position.
5. Repeat for the recommended amount of reps. The average is 8–12 repetitions.

EXERCISE 14

BICEP CURL

SCAN FOR VIDEO

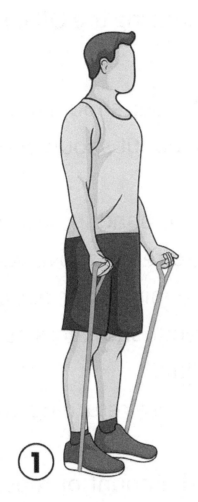
①

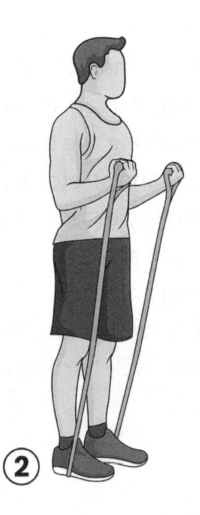
②

_*Upper Body Exercises | Exercise 14*

BICEP CURL

View a demo of this exercise by scanning the QR code or going to: primelifepress.com/rbub14

1. Begin by standing up tall with your shoulders down and back. Your feet should be underneath your hips.
2. Loop your resistance band underneath both of your feet and hold each end of the band in one hand with your palms facing forward. Let your arms hang by your side.
3. Bending at your elbows, slowly curl your hands up towards your shoulders while squeezing your biceps. Keep your elbows close to the sides of your body.
4. Lower your hands back to the starting position.
5. Repeat for the recommended amount of reps. The average is 15–20 repetitions.

BENT OVER REAR DELT FLY

SCAN FOR
VIDEO

①

②

BENT OVER REAR DELT FLY

View a demo of this exercise by scanning the QR code or going to: primelifepress.com/rbub15

1. Begin by standing up tall with your shoulders down and back. Your feet should be underneath your hips.
2. Loop your resistance band underneath both of your feet and hold each end of the band in one hand with your palms facing forward each other. You should be bending forward from your hips with your back straight.
3. Raise your arms straight out to your side until you reach shoulder height. Squeeze your shoulder blades together.
4. Lower your arms back to the starting position.
5. Repeat for the recommended amount of reps. The average is 10–12 repetitions.

EXERCISE 16
UPRIGHT ROW

SCAN FOR VIDEO

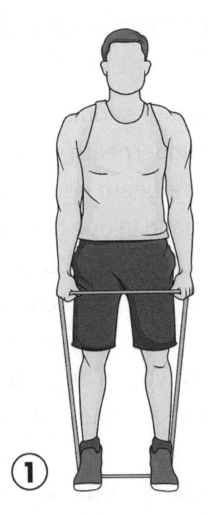

①

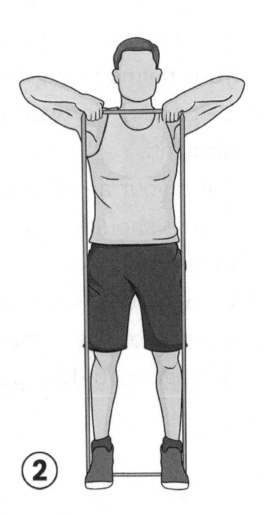

②

UPRIGHT ROW

View a demo of this exercise by scanning the QR code or going to: primelifepress.com/rbub16

1. Begin by standing up tall with your shoulders down and back. Your feet should be underneath your hips.
2. Loop your resistance band underneath both of your feet and hold each end of the band in one hand with your palms facing towards you.
3. Bending at the elbows, pull the band straight up the front of your body to shoulder level.
4. Slowly lower back to the starting position.
5. Repeat for the recommended amount of reps. The average is 10–12 repetitions.

BANDED SQUAT #1

SCAN FOR

VIDEO

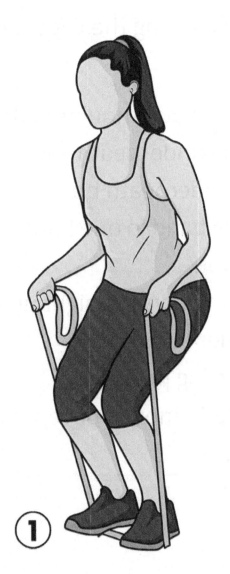

①

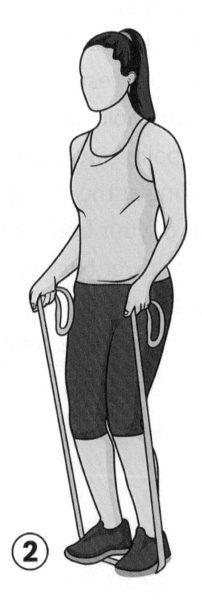

②

BANDED SQUAT #1

View a demo of this exercise by scanning the QR code or going to: primelifepress.com/rblb1

1. Begin by standing up tall with your shoulders back and down. Engage your core.
2. Place your feet shoulder-width apart with your toes turned slightly outwards.
3. Holding the end of the resistance band in each hand, loop it under both of your feet.
4. Create tension by pulling the band up towards the middle of your body.
5. Begin your squat by pushing your hips back and bending your knees as if you are sitting down.
6. Keep your back straight and your knees driving outwards, so they stay over your toes.
7. Stand up and return to your starting position.
8. Repeat for the recommended amount of reps. The average is 10–15 repetitions.

EXERCISE 18
BANDED SQUAT #2

SCAN FOR  VIDEO

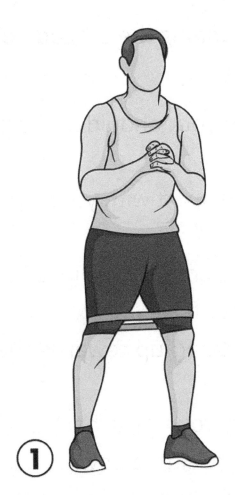

①

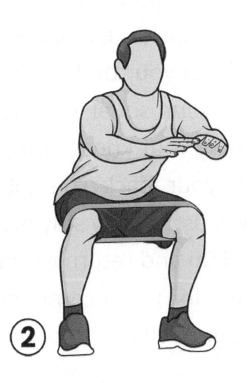

②

BANDED SQUAT #2

View a demo of this exercise by scanning the QR code or going to: primelifepress.com/rblb2

1. Begin by standing up tall with your shoulders back and down. Engage your core.
2. Place your resistance band above your knees.
3. Place your feet shoulder-width apart with your toes turned slightly outwards.
4. Begin your squat by pushing your hips back and bending your knees as if you are sitting down.
5. Keep your back straight and your knees driving outwards, so they stay over your toes.
6. Stand up and return to your starting position.
7. Repeat for the recommended amount of reps. The average is 10–15 repetitions.

EXERCISE 19
DEADLIFT

SCAN FOR

VIDEO

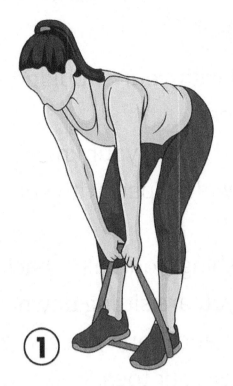

①

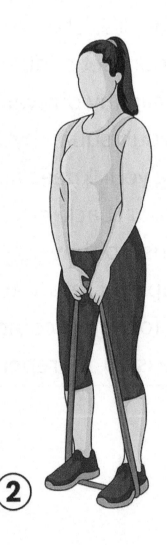

②

DEADLIFT

View a demo of this exercise by scanning the QR code or going to: primelifepress.com/rblb3

1. Begin by standing up tall with your shoulders down and back. Your feet should be placed hip distance apart.

2. Loop the resistance band underneath both feet and hold the other end with both hands.

3. Keep your arms straight and shift your hips backward into a hinge position.

4. Lower until your torso is parallel to the floor with your back straight.

5. Stand up straight, squeezing your glutes at the top.

6. Repeat for the recommended amount of reps. The average is 10–15 repetitions.

EXERCISE 20

KICKSTAND SINGLE LEG DEADLIFT

SCAN FOR VIDEO

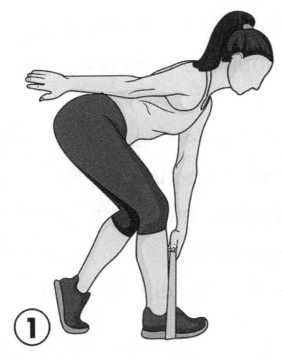

①

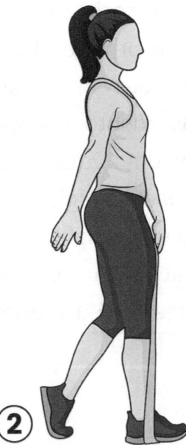

②

KICKSTAND SINGLE-LEG ROMANIAN DEADLIFT

View a demo of this exercise by scanning the QR code or going to: primelifepress.com/rblb4

1. Begin by standing up tall with your shoulders back and down.
2. Place your right foot in front of your left so that you are in a staggered stance. Keep your left foot resting on its ball. Widen your stance slightly if you feel off balance.
3. Holding the end of the resistance band in each hand, loop it under your right foot.
4. Bend your left leg slightly, engage your core, and bend forward from your hip while keeping your back straight. Keep tension on the band the entire time and you return to the starting position.
5. Repeat for the recommended amount of reps. The average is 10–15 repetitions.

EXERCISE 21

STANDING ADDUCTION

SCAN FOR VIDEO

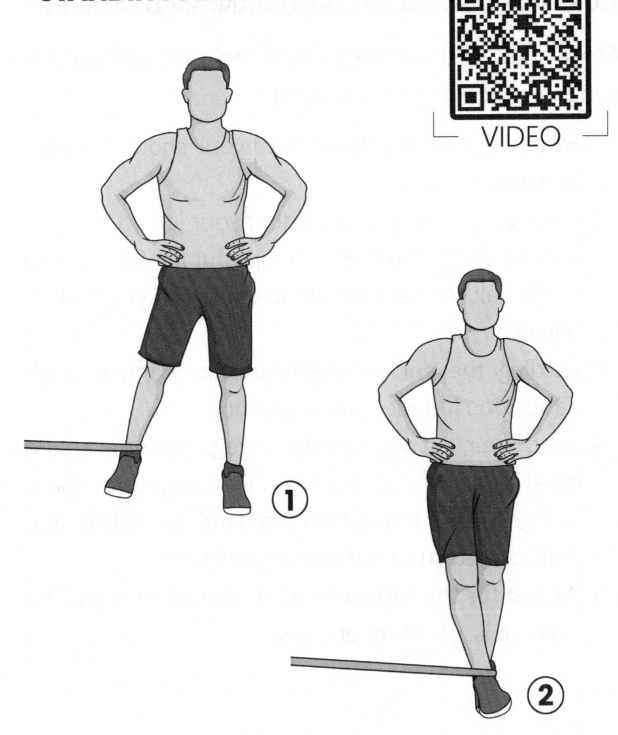

STANDING ADDUCTION

View a demo of this exercise by scanning the QR code or going to: primelifepress.com/rblb5

1. Anchor the resistance band at ankle height and stand tall in line with the band.
2. Wrap the free end of the band around your outer ankle.
3. Stand perpendicular to the band and create tension in the band by moving away from it.
4. From a wide stance, bend your knees slightly and get into a partial squat.
5. Pull your outer leg in toward your inner, working against the resistance.
6. Slowly return to the starting position.
7. Repeat for the recommended amount of reps. The average is 12–15 repetitions per side.

EXERCISE 22
LEG PRESS

SCAN FOR

VIDEO

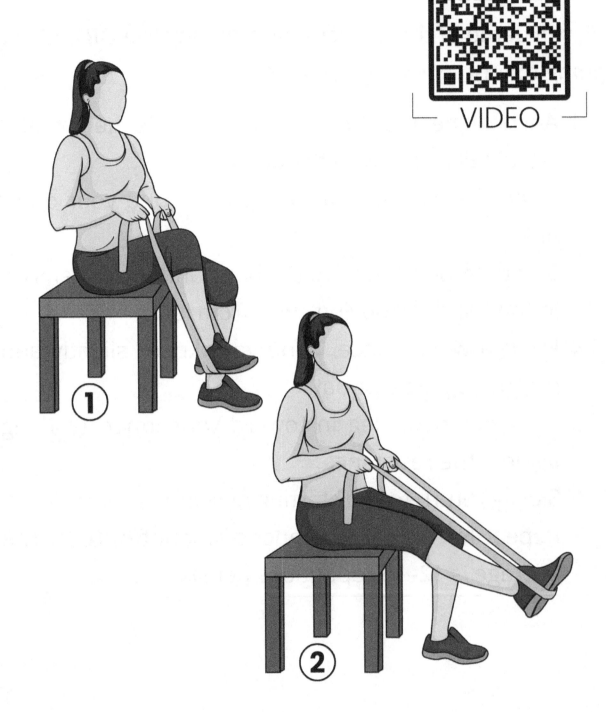

① ②

LEG PRESS

View a demo of this exercise by scanning the QR code or going to: primelifepress.com/rblb6

1. Begin by sitting upright in your chair with your shoulders down and back.
2. Hold both ends of the resistance band in your hands.
3. Place the band in the middle of the sole on your left foot.
4. Extend your leg out in front of you. Keep your right foot planted firmly on the ground.
5. Begin the movement by bending your left leg up towards your chest.
6. Extend it back to the starting position.
7. Repeat for the recommended amount of reps. The average is 10–15 repetitions per side.

CALF PRESS

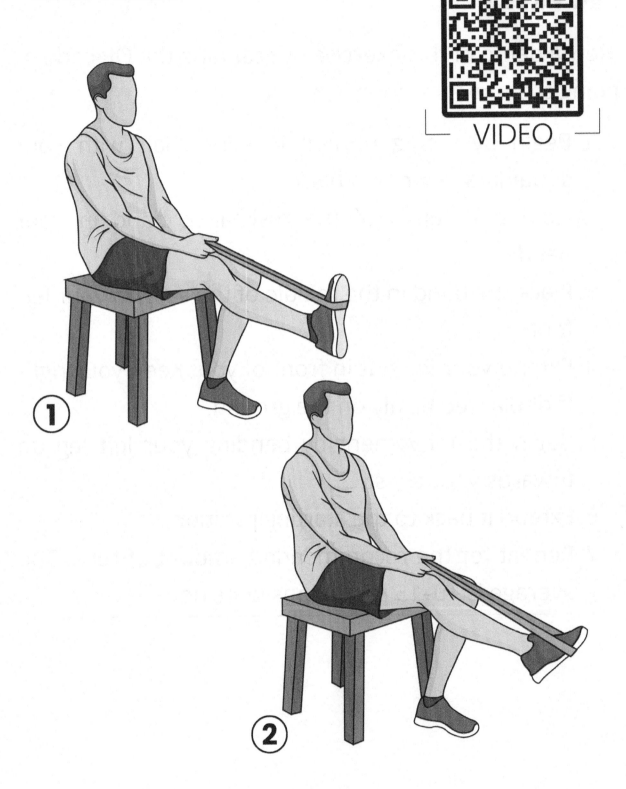

CALF PRESS

View a demo of this exercise by scanning the QR code or going to: primelifepress.com/rblb7

1. Begin by sitting upright in your chair with your shoulders down and back.
2. Hold both ends of the resistance band in your hands.
3. Place the band in the middle of the sole on your left foot.
4. Extend your leg out in front of you. Keep your right foot planted firmly on the ground.
5. Begin the movement by flexing your left foot forward toward the ground from the ankle.
6. Flex your toes upwards toward the ceiling.
7. Repeat for the recommended amount of reps. The average is 10–15 repetitions per side.

EXERCISE 24
LEG EXTENSION

SCAN FOR VIDEO

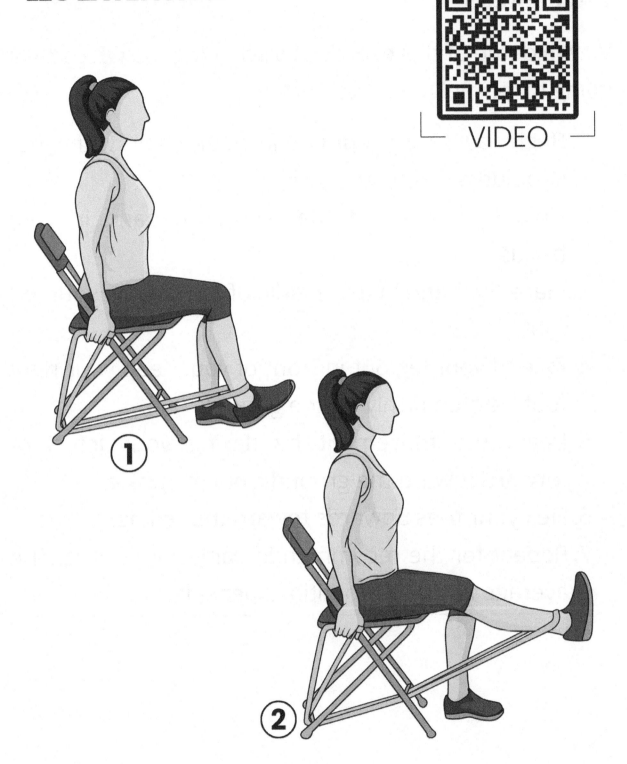

LEG EXTENSION

View a demo of this exercise by scanning the QR code or going to: primelifepress.com/rblb8

1. Begin by sitting upright in your chair with your shoulders down and back.
2. Place one end of the resistance band on the left back leg of your chair and the other end on your left ankle.
3. Keep both feet underneath your knees but create tension on the band so that it is slightly taut against your ankle.
4. Shift your weight to your right foot and lift your right leg from the floor.
5. Extend your knee until it straightens out in front of you.
6. Return to the starting position.
7. Repeat for the recommended amount of reps. The average is 8–12 repetitions per side.

EXERCISE 25
SITTING LEG CURL

SCAN FOR

VIDEO

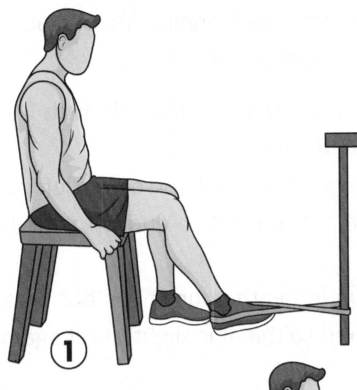

①

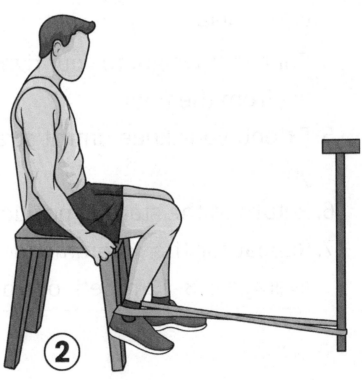

②

SITTING LEG CURL

View a demo of this exercise by scanning the QR code or going to: primelifepress.com/rblb9

1. Anchor the resistance band at a point that is close to the floor.
2. Sit in a chair, loop the band around your right ankle, and move away from the anchor so that the band becomes taut.
3. Bending at the knee, bring your right heel towards your glutes as far as you feel comfortable.
4. Return your leg to the starting position.
5. Repeat for the recommended amount of reps. The average is 10–15 repetitions per side.

EXERCISE 26
CLAMSHELLS

SCAN FOR
VIDEO

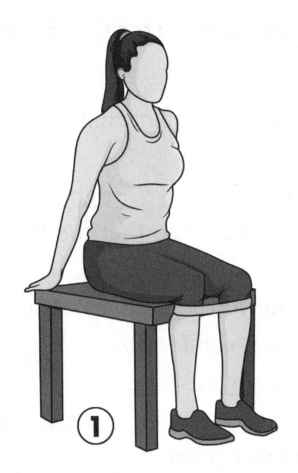

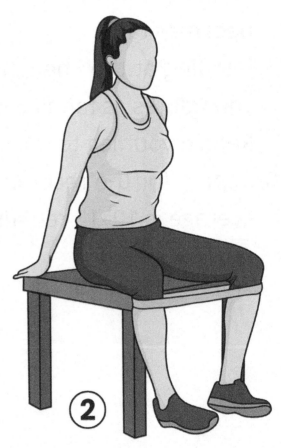

CLAMSHELLS

View a demo of this exercise by scanning the QR code or going to: primelifepress.com/rblb10

1. Loop a band around your legs just above your knees.
2. Sit in a chair or lie on the floor on your side, with one leg on top of the other and your knees slightly bent.
3. While keeping your feet together, pull your knees away from each other while squeezing your glutes for 2–3 seconds.
4. Slowly return to the starting position.
5. Repeat for the recommended amount of reps. The average is 10–12 repetitions per side.

BANDED LATERAL WALK

SCAN FOR VIDEO

① ② ③

BANDED LATERAL WALK

View a demo of this exercise by scanning the QR code or going to: primelifepress.com/rblb11

1. Begin by standing up tall with your shoulders back and down. Engage your core.
2. Your feet should be hip-width apart.
3. Place a band around the top of your ankles.
4. Bend slightly at your knees into a partial squat.
5. Step to the right with your right foot.
6. Follow with your left foot so that you return to the middle with your feet hip-width apart.
7. Repeat for the recommended amount of reps and then swap sides. The average is 10–15 repetitions per side.

EXERCISE 28
GLUTE BRIDGE

SCAN FOR VIDEO

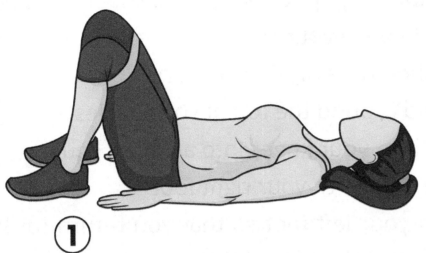

①

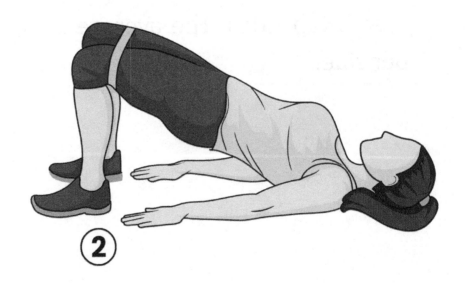

②

GLUTE BRIDGE

View a demo of this exercise by scanning the QR code or going to: primelifepress.com/rblb12

1. Begin by lying flat on your back.
2. Place the resistance band above your knees and place your feet flat on the floor with your knees at 90° and your heels placed just outside your glutes.
3. Lift your hips by contracting your glutes.
4. As you raise them, apply outward pressure from your knees against the band.
5. Repeat for the recommended amount of reps. The average is 15–20 repetitions.

EXERCISE 29
PALLOF PRESS

SCAN FOR
VIDEO

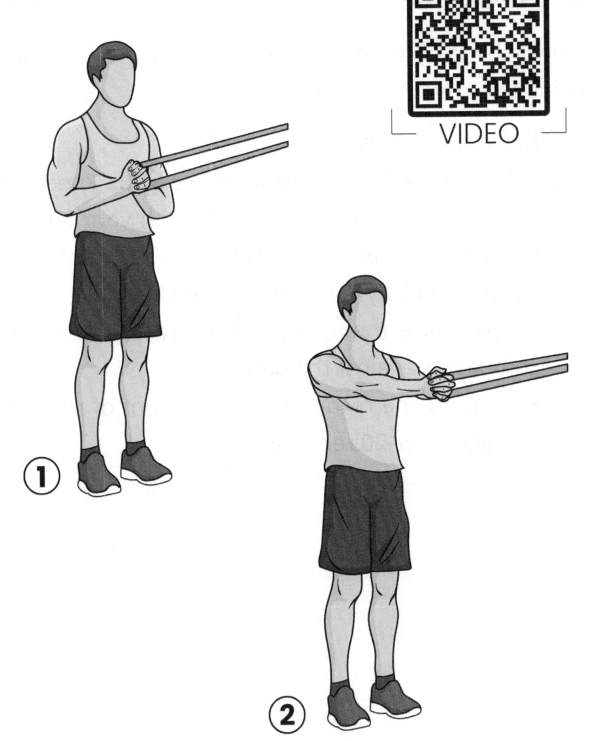

PALLOF PRESS

View a demo of this exercise by scanning the QR code or going to: primelifepress.com/rbfb1

1. Sit tall in a chair next to a door or anchor point where you will anchor your resistance band.
2. Anchor your band so that it is chest height.
3. Hold the resistance band in both hands and position yourself so that there is tension on the band, and it is slightly pulling you towards the anchor point.
4. Place your knees shoulder-width apart and hold the handle with your hands in front of you.
5. Brace your core and slowly press your hands in front of you until they are straight.
6. Pause for a second and return them to your chest.
7. Repeat for the recommended amount of reps and then swap sides. The average is 8–12 repetitions per side.

EXERCISE 30
WOODCHOPPER

SCAN FOR

VIDEO

①

②

WOODCHOPPER

View a demo of this exercise by scanning the QR code or going to: primelifepress.com/rbfb2

1. Anchor the band close to the floor on a stable and secure object.
2. Move the chair so that there is the required amount of resistance at the starting position. Keep your chest up and core activated.
3. Keep your arms straight and hanging down towards your left foot.
4. Pull the band diagonally upwards towards the right and straighten it out to the overhead in a chopping motion. Your hip will gently twist as you raise upwards, and your left foot will pivot as well.
5. Lower your arms back to the starting position.
6. Repeat for the recommended amount of reps and then swap sides. The average is 8–10 repetitions per side.

EXERCISE 31

ANTI-ROTATION BAND WALKOUT

SCAN FOR

VIDEO

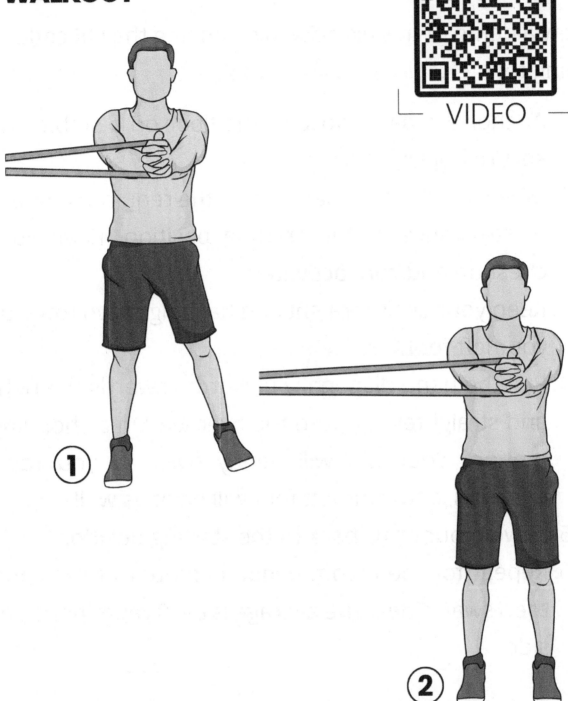

① ②

ANTI-ROTATION BAND WALKOUT

View a demo of this exercise by scanning the QR code or going to: primelifepress.com/rbfb3

1. Begin by anchoring your band to a door or pillar at chest height.
2. Keeping the band to the outside of your body, hold onto the other end with both hands.
3. Move away from the anchor point to create tension in the band.
4. Bend your knees slightly and get into a partial squat.
5. Hold the band with both hands straight out in front of your chest and step sideways away from the band until it is too tense to go any further.
6. Slowly move back toward the anchor point to the starting position.
7. Repeat for the recommended amount of reps and then swap sides. The average is 6–8 repetitions per side.

RUSSIAN TWIST

SCAN FOR
VIDEO

①

②

RUSSIAN TWIST

View a demo of this exercise by scanning the QR code or going to: primelifepress.com/rbfb4

1. Begin by sitting tall in your chair with your legs out in front of you with a bend in your knee.
2. Loop the center of the band around the soles of your feet and hold the other end of your band with both hands.
3. Gently lean back at a 45° angle, keeping your arms straight in front of you and in line with your chest.
4. Keeping the back of your heels on the floor, rotate from your hips towards your right side, bringing your hands to just outside your right hip.
5. Rotate to the left side. That is one repetition.
6. Repeat for the recommended amount of reps. The average is 10–12 repetitions.

BANDED BICYCLE CRUNCH

SCAN FOR VIDEO

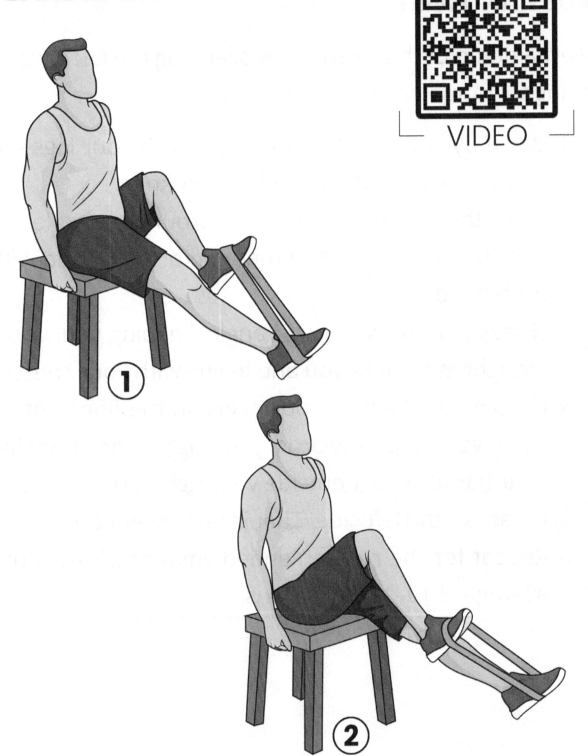

BANDED BICYCLE CRUNCH

View a demo of this exercise by scanning the QR code or going to: primelifepress.com/rbfb5

1. Begin by sitting up tall in your chair.
2. Loop a short band around your feet, place your hands behind your butt and lean back at 45 degrees.
3. Push out with your right foot and pull in with your left.
4. Swap sides and do the same on the other side.
5. Repeat for the recommended amount of reps. The average is 10–12 repetitions per side.

BANDED BIRD DOG

SCAN FOR VIDEO

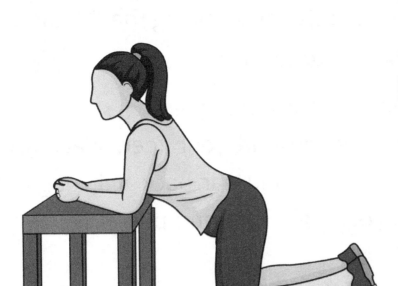

①

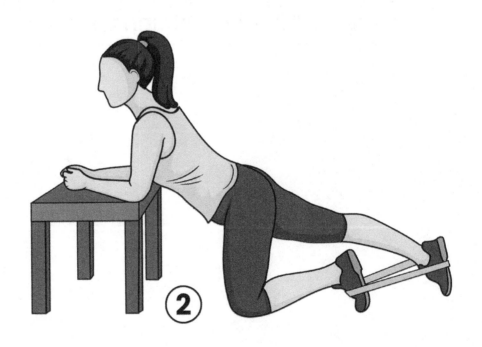

②

BANDED BIRD DOG

View a demo of this exercise by scanning the QR code or going to: primelifepress.com/rbfb6

1. Begin on all fours with your knees underneath your hips and your palms underneath your shoulders. Keep your back straight and your midline engaged.
2. Place your resistance band on both feet at the arches.
3. Extend your left leg out straight behind you and just barely touch you left toe to the floor.
4. Pull your left leg back and set your knee on the floor then do the same with the right leg.
5. Repeat this movement for the recommended amount of reps. The average is 8–12 repetitions per side.

EXERCISE 35

PENGUIN CRUNCH

SCAN FOR

VIDEO

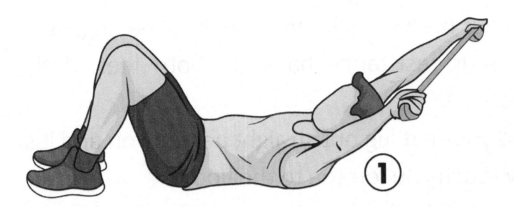

①

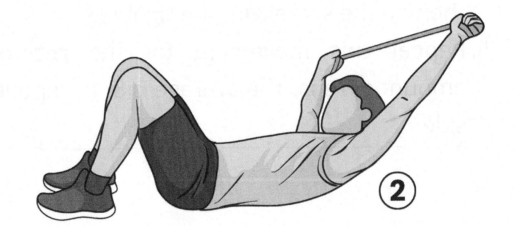

②

PENGUIN CRUNCH

View a demo of this exercise by scanning the QR code or going to: primelifepress.com/rbfb7

1. Begin by lying on your back, holding the ends of the resistance band in each hand. Keep the band taut.
2. Bend your knees and keep your feet flat on the floor. Slowly raise your shoulders off the ground slightly.
3. Extend your arms overhead.
4. Crunch your torso towards the right and return to the center.
5. Crunch your torso towards the left and return to the center.
6. Repeat this movement for the recommended amount of reps. The average is 8–12 repetitions per side.

EXERCISE 36
DONKEY KICK

SCAN FOR

VIDEO

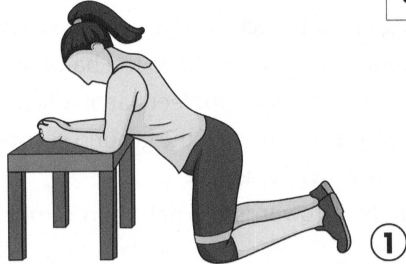

①

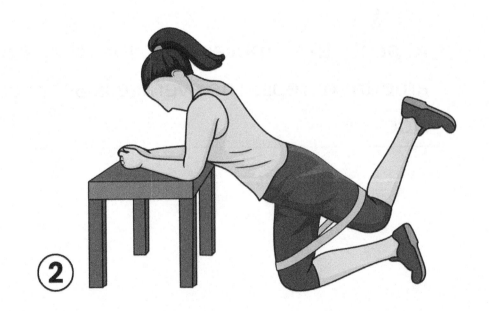

②

DONKEY KICK

View a demo of this exercise by scanning the QR code or going to: primelifepress.com/rbfb8

1. Begin on all fours, with your knees underneath your hips and your palms underneath your shoulders. Keep your back straight and your midline engaged.
2. Place your resistance band around your thighs, just above the knee.
3. Raise your right leg off the floor and kick your right foot up toward the ceiling.
4. Keep your leg in line with your hip.
5. Return your leg to the starting position
6. Swap legs.
7. Repeat this movement for the recommended amount of reps. The average is 8–12 repetitions per side.

Repetition and Set Recommendations for Different Fitness Levels

You now have a comprehensive exercise library, and soon you will have a workout that you can perform as well. But before we continue we need to talk about frequency, volume, and intensity.

What does that mean? It means how often you should train, how many exercises, sets, and reps you should do, and how hard it should be.

When you put together your workouts, these are things you will need to take into consideration.

How Often Should You Train?

According to Colberg (2017), you should aim to do some form of resistance training at least two times a week, but it would be preferable to do three.

These should be nonconsecutive days which will allow your muscles to rest and recover for your next session. You do not want to work the same muscle groups daily as this hinders recovery and our muscles do not repair themselves—it is when we recover that we get stronger.

If you do want to do resistance training for three days a week, you should alternate muscle groups. Alternatively, you can rest a day in between each training session.

An example of a weekly workout routine could look like the following:

If you are just starting, you could allocate two days per week to exercising, where you will work out on Monday and Thursday. You would stick to this for four to six weeks. Remember to be consistent, as consistency is the key to getting the results you are after.

Once you have completed four to six weeks of training, you can move to three days a week, training Monday, Wednesday, and Thursday. Allowing a day in between workouts.

It is important to remember that even if you are starting and can only manage one day a week, you will still reap the benefits that strength training provides.

How Many Movements, Sets, and Reps Should You Be Doing?

This depends on how many times a week you work out, what muscles you use, and how intense the workout is.

The general recommendation is to aim for about six movements per workout that work a range of muscle groups—upper, lower, and core.

When it comes to sets, you should work with one to three sets per movement, with anything from three to 20 repetitions per set. A good general guideline is to start with 8 to 12 repetitions and two to three sets, with rest in the middle of each set as needed.

Start very conservatively with low reps and low resistance, and gradually work your way up to more reps and higher resistance. A basic strength progression using progressive overload could look like this.

In week one, you perform one set of your movements, doing eight reps a set. The next week, you do the same, but you work up to 20 reps. On week three, you use a slightly heavier band and you do 12 repetitions.

There are also other ways to progress and get stronger that do not necessarily mean more resistance or more repetitions. You can increase the difficulty of your workout by doing more challenging exercises, decreasing the time that you rest in between your sets, or even adding another set.

Play around and get creative with the way you structure your program, but always listen to your body.

Remember to also include your warm-up cool-downs in your workout sessions.

To sum it up:

- Get the all-clear from your doctor.
- Stop exercising if you begin to feel dizzy, such as unusual shortness of breath, chest discomfort, palpitations, or joint pain.
- Initially aim for one to two sessions a week with six exercises to start.
- Once you are comfortable and your fitness levels improve, add another day to your program.
- Work towards two to three sets per exercise, 10 to 15 reps to start.
- Do not work the same muscles on consecutive days.
- Increase weights over time.

Remember that these are general guidelines and everyone has a different fitness level and needs, which will change the guidelines. The key is to experiment, note how you perform and feel, and adjust accordingly.

When Will You Start Seeing Results?

You may not be seeing them or feeling them, but you have already improved but starting to exercise and doing one workout. If you work hard, eat well, sleep well, and manage your stress (more about these in the later chapters), you can start noticing progress as early as one or two weeks into your routine.

As a beginner to exercise, your body and brain are busy forming new connections and reactivating your motor units which may have been lying dormant due to inactivity (Kutcher, 2019). They are now being recruited whenever you do your strength training and are being conditioned to get stronger to complete the tasks you are asking them to do.

If you are looking to increase your muscle mass, this takes a while longer to accomplish. Once again you need to make sure you are eating well, sleeping well, and managing any stresses, but if you are consistent in these areas as well as with your strength training you may begin to notice a difference in four to six weeks.

This is known as hypertrophy, where your muscles begin to grow. If you have previously worked out or played sports you may find that due to muscle memory, this may occur faster and easier.

Chapter 6: Resistance Band Workouts

The following chapter will provide you with a few resistance band workouts that you can follow as you become more comfortable with the movements. You can use these as a template and swap out certain exercises, add sets and repetitions, or you can follow them as is. I will provide simple upper body, lower body, and full body workouts.

You can find all the movements in Chapter 5 and the warm-up and cool-down movements in Chapter 3.

EXERCISE 37
UPPER BODY : WORKOUT 1

SCAN FOR VIDEO

①

②

③

④

⑤

⑥

UPPER BODY WORKOUT ONE

View a demo of this workout by scanning the QR code or going to: primelifepress.com/woup1

Warm-Up

Complete two rounds of the following warm-up:

- 30 seconds of marching
- 10-12 neck rotations
- 10 shoulder rolls
- 10 arm circles
- 10 T-arm rotations

Work-Out

- 1 set of 8 banded pull apart
- 1 set of 10 upright rows
- 1 set of 8 overhead press
- 1 set of 10 chest press
- 1 set of 15 bicep curls
- 1 set of 10 cuff pivot

Cool-Down:

- 1 minute of slow marching
- 30 seconds bicep and shoulder stretch
- 30 seconds chest opener

UPPER BODY : WORKOUT 2

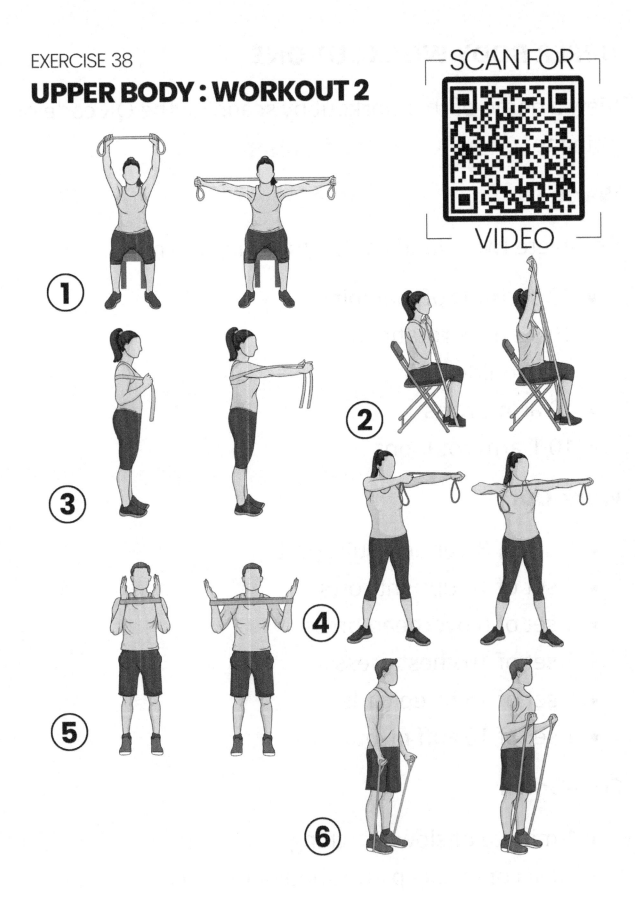

UPPER BODY WORKOUT TWO

View a demo of this workout by scanning the QR code or going to: primelifepress.com/woup2

Warm-Up

Complete **two** rounds of the following warm-up:

- 30 seconds of shadowboxing
- 10-12 head rolls
- 10 forearm circles
- 10 arm circles
- 10 bow and bends

Work-Out

- 1 set of 8 overhead pull apart
- 1 set of 8 overhead press
- 1 set of 10 chest press
- 1 set of 1 bow and arrow
- 1 set of 10 scapular retraction
- 1 set of 10 bicep curls

Cool-Down:

- 1 minute of slow marching
- 10 cat/cow
- 30 seconds chest opener
- 30 seconds overhead stretch

UPPER BODY : WORKOUT 3

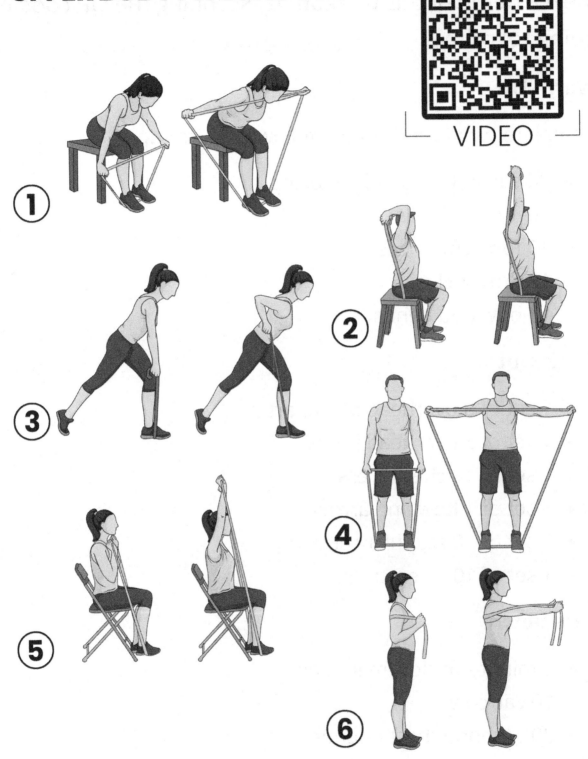

UPPER BODY WORKOUT THREE

View a demo of this workout by scanning the QR code or going to: primelifepress.com/woup3

Warm-Up

Complete **two** rounds of the following warm-up:

- 30 seconds of box-stepping
- 10 neck lateral flexion
- 10 wrist rotations
- 10 cats/cows

Work-Out

- 1 set of 10 bent-over rear delt fly
- 1 set of 10 overhead tricep extension
- 1 set of 10 staggered stance row
- 1 set of 1 banded lateral raise
- 1 set of 10 overhead press
- 1 set of 10 chest press

Cool-Down

- 1 minute of slow box stepping
- 30 seconds tricep stretch
- 30 seconds chest opener

EXERCISE 40
LOWER BODY : WORKOUT 1

SCAN FOR VIDEO

①

②

③

④

⑤

⑥

LOWER BODY WORKOUT ONE

View a demo of this workout by scanning the QR code or going to: primelifepress.com/wolb1

Warm-Up

Complete **two** rounds of the following warm-up:

- 30 seconds of lateral side steps
- 10 bows and bends
- 10 leg swings
- 10 thoracic rotation

Work-Out

- 1 set of 10 banded squat #1
- 1 set of 10 standing adduction
- 1 set of 10 leg press
- 1 set of 10 calf press
- 1 set of 10 glute bridges
- 1 set of 10 leg extension

Cool-Down

- 1 minute of slow lateral side steps
- 10 cat/cow
- 10 adductor stretch

LOWER BODY : WORKOUT 2

SCAN FOR VIDEO

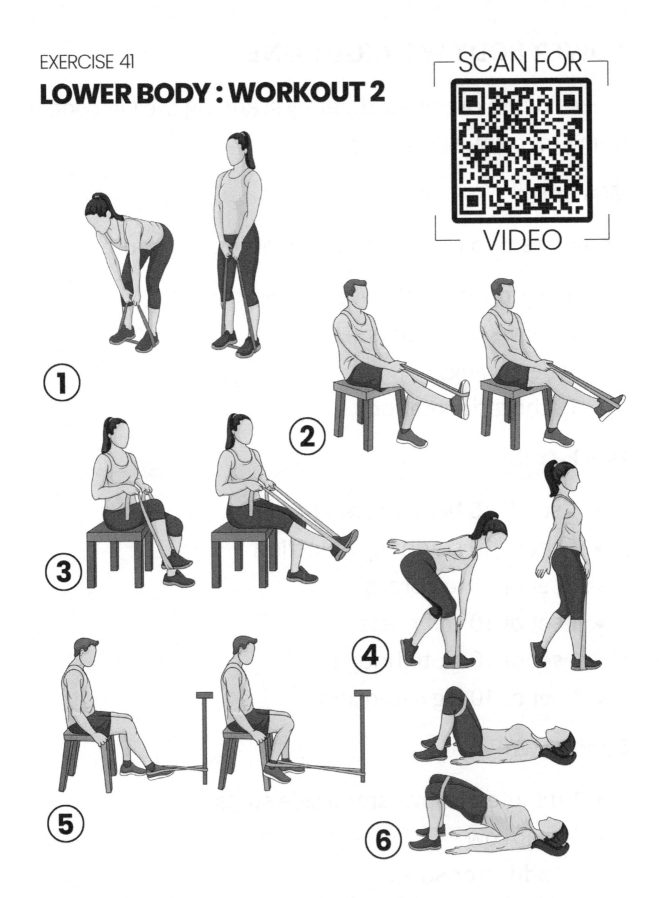

LOWER BODY WORKOUT TWO

View a demo of this workout by scanning the QR code or going to: primelifepress.com/wolb2

Warm-Up

Complete **two** rounds of the following warm-up:

- 30 seconds of butt kicks
- 10 cat/cow
- 10 hip rotations
- 10 ankle circles

Work-Out

- 1 set of 10 deadlift
- 1 set of 10 leg press
- 1 set of 10 calf press
- 1 set of 10 kickstand single-leg Romanian deadlift
- 1 set of 10 sitting leg curls
- 1 set of 10 glute bridges

Cool-Down

- 1 minute of slow butt kicks
- 30 seconds hamstring stretch
- 30 seconds hip lateral rotation

EXERCISE 42

LOWER BODY : WORKOUT 3

SCAN FOR VIDEO

①
②
③
④
⑤
⑥

LOWER BODY WORKOUT THREE

View a demo of this workout by scanning the QR code or going to: primelifepress.com/wolb3

Warm-Up

Complete **two** rounds of the following warm-up:

- 30 seconds of toe taps
- 10 leg swings
- 10 bow and bends
- 10 ankle circles

Work-Out

- 1 set of 10 clamshells
- 1 set of 10 standing adductors
- 1 set of 10 banded squat #2
- 1 set of 10 kickstand single-leg Romanian deadlift
- 1 set of 10 banded lateral walks
- 1 set of 10 calf press

Cool-Down

- 1 minute of slow butt kicks
- 30 seated hip flexions
- 30 seconds hamstring stretch

EXERCISE 43
FULL BODY : WORKOUT 1

SCAN FOR VIDEO

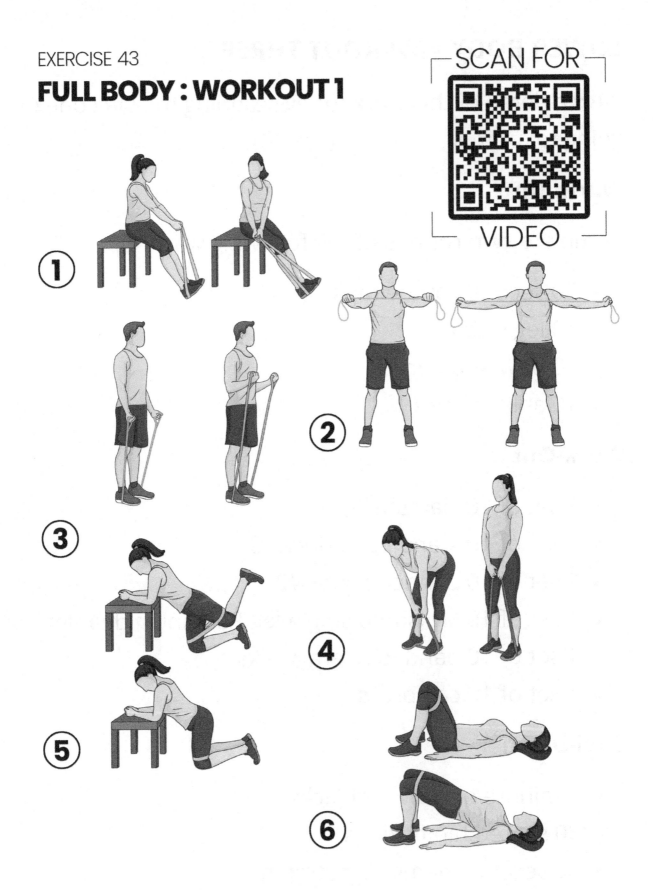

FULL BODY WORKOUT ONE

View a demo of this workout by scanning the QR code or going to: primelifepress.com/wofb1

Warm-Up

Complete **two** rounds of the following warm-up:

- 30 seconds of knees to elbows marching
- 10 head rolls
- 10 arm circles
- 10 leg swings

Work-Out

- 1 set of 10 Russian twists
- 1 set of 10 bands pull apart
- 1 set of 10 bicep curls
- 1 set of 10 deadlifts
- 1 set of 10 donkey kicks
- 1 set of 10 glute bridges

Cool-Down

- 1 minute of slow knees-to-elbows marching
- 30-second quad stretch
- 30 seconds hamstring stretch

FULL BODY : WORKOUT 2

SCAN FOR VIDEO

①

②

③

④

⑤

⑥

FULL BODY WORKOUT TWO

View a demo of this workout by scanning the QR code or going to: primelifepress.com/wofb2

Warm-Up

Complete **two** rounds of the following warm-up:

- 30 seconds of shuffle steps
- 10 wrist rotations
- 10 forearm circles
- 10 bows and bends

Work-Out

- 1 set of 10 Pallof press
- 1 set of 10 banded bicycle crunches
- 1 set of 10 banded bird dogs
- 1 set of 10 donkey kicks
- 1 set of 10 leg press
- 1 set of 10 chest press

Cool-Down

- 1 minute of slow shuffle steps
- 30 second lower back stretch
- 30 seconds seated hip flexion

EXERCISE 45

FULL BODY : WORKOUT 3

SCAN FOR VIDEO

①
②
③
④
⑤
⑥

FULL BODY WORKOUT THREE

View a demo of this workout by scanning the QR code or going to: primelifepress.com/wofb3

Warm-Up

Complete **two** rounds of the following warm-up:

- 30 seconds of heel digs
- 10 shoulder rolls
- 10 arm circles
- 10 cat/cow

Work-Out

- 1 set of 10 overhead press
- 1 set of 10 chest press
- 1 set of 10 penguin crunches
- 1 set of 10 woodchoppers
- 1 set of 10 banded squat #2
- 1 set of 10 banded lateral walks

Cool-Down

- 1 minute of slow heel digs
- 30-second lumbar side stretch

Chapter 7: Lifestyle and Wellbeing

You now have all the relevant knowledge that you need to confidently start your exercise routine, but that is often easier said than done.

By following our tips in Chapter 2 you can confidently begin your journey to wellness and longevity, but do you know there is more to it than just exercise? I want you to achieve holistic wellness, which means other pillars of health may need some attention. These being

- nutrition
- stress
- sleep

You need to make sure that you eat enough nutritious food to keep your energy levels up and provide you with enough nutrients and minerals to keep you healthy. You also need to make sure that you are sufficiently hydrated.

Sleep is very important in managing our health. Lack of sleep can put us at risk of getting sick.

Long-term stress can also impact our health and put us at risk for various diseases and disorders.

This chapter will look at these three additional pillars of health and how you can optimize them on your journey to holistic health.

Nutrition

As we age, our needs change due to a certain number of factors. Our protein requirements increase, our calorie needs may decrease, we may need more vitamins such as calcium, and we may need more fiber. Let's look at some of the changes we will need to navigate as we get older. Remember, we want to eat well, so we can exercise and stay as healthy as possible.

Lower Calorie Intake

As you get older, and become less active, you may need to lower your calorie intake, but at the same time, you may need more nutritionally dense food.

As we age, our bodies may have difficulty absorbing certain nutrients, or we may just need more of them to maintain our health. Calcium and vitamin D are two nutrients that come to mind.

Calcium becomes more difficult to absorb as we age, and it is believed that this can be a knock-on result of not getting enough vitamin D (Raman, 2017). You may need to increase your intake of both vitamins as you get older to ensure you are reaching your recommended daily requirements. You could either do this by eating food that is high in each vitamin or using supplements.

In addition to calcium and vitamin D, vitamin B12 levels should be tested, as this is another vitamin that becomes difficult to absorb. We can get B12 from eggs, fish meat, or dairy, but if needed you can get it in supplement form as well.

Appetite Changes

You may be experiencing a decrease in you are appetite. This poses a problem as you may find yourself not consuming enough calories to meet your energy requirements, or you may not get the right amount of nutrients, vitamins, and minerals that your body needs to function optimally.

This occurs due to the changes in our hormones, with hunger hormones declining and fullness hormones increasing. Our sense of taste and smell also changes as the years go, by which may make food unappealing (Raman, 2017).

Counter this by experimenting with eating smaller meals throughout the day or including more snacks in your diet plan.

Protein Needs Increase

Due to the loss of muscle and the difficulty your body has in maintaining and building it, it is advised that we raise our protein intake to ensure we are getting enough to lessen the risk of sarcopenia.

Eating more protein or supplementing with protein can reduce the risk of strength loss and even help build more muscle, keeping us strong as we age.

Fiber Becomes a Focus

Finding it difficult to go to the toilet regularly is a common complaint as the years go on. It is a common problem in those over 60, especially women.

There are two reasons that this may occur. The first is that we tend to move less, and we may be taking medication that can add to the problem. Exercise is a good tool for preventing and relieving constipation, as is increasing your fiber intake.

Now that you are aware of the common nutritional changes that occur as we get older, you can begin to structure your diet to prevent and address them.

According to Healthy Eating Tips for Seniors (2021), there are several tips that when followed can help get or keep your nutrition on track.

- Identify what a healthy, balanced meal looks like.
- Know your nutrients and eat a variety of different foods to get the recommended amount.
- Learn how to read nutritional labels.
- Familiarize yourself with how recommended servings work.
- Stay hydrated.

What Does a Balanced Meal Consist Of?

According to What Is MyPlate? (2020) there are specific dietary needs that older adults have as they age. We need to ensure that we eat a variety of different foods to ensure we obtain the nutrients, vitamins, and minerals that we need to reduce the risk of developing chronic diseases and ailments. As we age, we are more at risk of developing diabetes, high blood pressure, hypertension, and cardiovascular disease.

Additionally, while adding a range of healthy food, we need to limit our intake of saturated fat, sugar, and sodium.

We need to be aware of eating the right amount of food for our activity levels so that we can maintain a healthy body weight. It is suggested that we focus on our protein intake and ensure we are eating enough of this macronutrient to maintain our muscle mass.

As we age, we also lose our sense of thirst, and we may inadvertently drink less water than we need. Counteract this by drinking water often, drinking a glass at every meal when you wake up, and sipping on it throughout the day.

So what does a healthy, balanced meal look like? According to What Is MyPlate? (2020) Protein should make up a ¼ of your plate, vegetables should make up another ¼ of your plate, fruit should make up slightly less than ¼ of your plate and grains should make up the rest. You should aim for one serving of dairy per meal.

When it comes to fruit, focus on whole fruits. They can be fresh, frozen, canned, or even dried. To add more fruit to your diet, make them easily available on your kitchen counter and use them as snacks throughout the day.

When it comes to vegetables, I like to say that you should be eating the rainbow, meaning that you should eat a wide variety of vegetables in all different colors. Add them to stews, casseroles, wraps, and even sandwiches. Like fruit, they can be frozen, canned, or fresh.

When it comes to grains, aim to eat whole-grain versions of rice, pasta, and bread or tortillas. They provide more fiber, nutrients, and minerals than their counterparts.

You should aim to eat lean protein from both animal sources and plant sources. Plant sources include beans, legumes, and soy. Animal-based protein comes from lean pieces of meat, seafood, poultry, and nuts and seeds.

For your serving of dairy, it is recommended that you choose fat-free or low-fat versions. This will help you reach your calcium needs.

How to Read Food Labels

Knowing what you are consuming empowers you to make better food choices. Learning to read a nutrition label can help you make healthier choices when presented with processed foods.

You will find the total number of servings at the top of the label. This tells you the total number of portions that are in the container and the food serving size. The serving size is not the recommendation of how much you should eat, rather, it is the amount of food that people may eat at one time.

The following information on the label will be based on the single serving size.

The Daily Value is based on a 2,000-calorie diet and refers to how much a nutrient in that serving of food contributes to the diet.

The ingredient list is usually found underneath the nutrition facts label. It lists the ingredients in descending order by their weight. The largest ingredient is listed first. Look out for the following ingredients, as these are added sugars:

- brown sugar
- corn sweetener
- corn syrup
- dextrose
- fructose
- high-fructose corn syrup (How to Read Food and Beverage Labels, 2022)

You may also see labels such as *organic, light, low,* or *reduced*. Usually, these are clever marketing terms that give us the impression that the food is healthy, when in most cases it has no bearing on the nutritional quality.

How Much Water Should I Drink?

Dehydration can be a risk as we get older. According to How to Stay Hydrated for Better Health (2021), we are more prone to becoming dehydrated due to our appetite and thirst diminishing as we age—our body's signals do not work as effectively. Additionally, we may be taking medication that can reduce our thirst.

The general rule for water intake is to take one-third of your body weight and drink that amount in ounces.

Discuss this with your doctor, as there are special circumstances where you may need a more tailored approach to your water intake.

If you are looking to increase your fluid intake, there are some simple things you can do to add more fluid to your diet.

You can include water-rich foods in your meals. Cucumbers, watermelon, lettuce, tomatoes, celery, and lettuce are foods that are high in water content and can contribute to your daily intake. Soups and broths are also good options, just opt for low-sodium options.

Get yourself a glass water bottle and keep it with you so you can sip on it throughout the day.

Alcohol, being a diuretic, triggers your body to remove fluid from your bloodstream. Reduce or avoid alcohol, as this will help your body hold on to more moisture.

Stress

Stress occurs when our reactions to certain circumstances are challenging to regulate and control. Essentially it is a mental reaction to distressing situations such as losing your job, getting older, or any other significant life-affecting events (*Stress and How to Reduce It: A Guide for Older Adults*, n.d.).

Stress is a normal part of life; in small doses, it is healthy. Stress has developed as an evolutionary response that helps keep us safe by initiating our *fight-or-flight* responses.

Stress manifests either physically or mentally, and it has become such a common aspect of our lives that it is often hard for us to notice we may be suffering from chronic stress.

According to *Stress and How to Reduce It: A Guide for Older Adults* (n.d.), stress may affect older adults more than their younger counterparts.

Stress causes inflammation in the body and inflammation is one of the root causes of certain diseases, therefore, when we are stressed, we are more likely to be at risk of certain diseases or our symptoms may worsen. Diseases that pose the most risk when stressed are arthritis, atherosclerosis, dementia, cancer, and type 2 diabetes.

If you are going through some of the following situations, you may be under stress and unaware:

- significant life changes, such as retirement
- illness
- death and grief
- loneliness
- financial difficulties
- increased responsibilities

If you are going through one of the life events, pay attention to the cues your body may be giving you, There are subtle symptoms of stress that we often neglect as we go about daily life.

- low mood
- irritability
- headaches
- racing heart
- digestive problems
- sleep issues
- lack of focus
- isolation

These are just general examples, and you may exhibit stress in different ways, it is important to listen to your body and identify if anything seems off or different for you.

Tips for Managing Stress

Simple changes to your lifestyle can help you manage your stress and get you on the path to holistic wellness. Pick one or two of these strategies and implement them over the next couple of weeks.

Remove the Source

This is sometimes easier said than done, but the first solution you should explore is removing the source of your stress. If that is impossible, reach out and ask for help. Take small steps to help alleviate any of the burden you are experiencing.

Exercise

You are already on the path to responsibly managing your stress by beginning this exercise program. You are aware of the health benefits of exercise in terms of the physical effects it can have, now you can add mental benefits to that list as well.

Nourish Yourself Well

Pay attention to your diet and ensure that you are eating well. A balanced, varied, and nutritionally packed diet helps lift your mood, improve your immune system, and reduce inflammation. It will provide more energy and enhance your feeling of well-being.

Get Quality Sleep

Sleep allows our bodies to rest and recover and has proven to have a significant impact on our physical and mental well-being. We will discuss sleep in further detail later on in this chapter.

Stay Hydrated

Along with nutrition, you should pay attention to how much water you consume and make sure that you are sufficiently hydrated. Water keeps headaches at bay and improves cognitive function. It plays a significant role in digestion, and cognitive ability and can boost your energy. The bottom line is that drinking enough water makes you feel good.

Practice Mindfulness

Whether you meditate, practice breathing exercises, do yoga, or practice visualization, mindfulness can be a great tool for reducing stress. The effects have been well-researched and include lowering heart rate, calming anxiety, relaxing our nervous system and muscles, and creating a sense of peace, calm, and acceptance.

Take some time to find a way to practice mindfulness in a way that works for you. Journaling, meditation, walking in nature—there are many ways to reconnect with yourself and ease your mind.

Conclusion

I applaud you. It is not easy to start a journey towards better health and vitality from scratch. Well done for taking your health into your own hands and embracing exercise—you have taken an important step that is going to provide you with a new quality of life as well as create a new wonderful outlook.

Through some determination and commitment, you will prove that age is not a barrier to achieving strength, flexibility, and overall well-being.

As we have explored the countless benefits of resistance band exercises throughout this book, it is evident that you have the power to transform your life through simple yet effective workouts. By incorporating these exercises into your daily routines, you are not only improving your physical health, but also enhancing your mental and emotional well-being.

Remember that each stretch, each rep, and each moment of pushing beyond your comfort zone is a testament to your resilience and determination. It is only making you healthier and giving you the vitality and longevity you deserve.

The same principles apply to your nutrition, sleep, and stress management. These pillars of health should also be attended to to create holistic wellness. I am certain that as you get deeper into your healthy lifestyle, these aspects will all line up and fall into place together.

Your commitment to your well-being is an inspiration. Remember, it's never too late to start, and with each workout and each healthy meal, you are rewriting the narrative of aging.

As you continue on this path, may you find strength in every challenge, joy in every achievement, and a renewed sense of vitality that empowers you to live life to the fullest.

Keep moving and keep believing in the incredible potential within you. The best is yet to come!

References

Acosta, K. (2021, August 4). How your posture affects your health. Forbes Health. https://www.forbes.com/health/body/how-to-fix-bad-posture/

American Psychological Association. (2021, September). Older adults' health and age-related changes. https://www.apa.org. https://www.apa.org/pi/aging/resources/guides/older

Ayuda, T. (2021, July 31). 6 resistance band exercises that will smoke your entire upper body. SELF. https://www.self.com/gallery/upper-body-circuit-workout-resistance-bands

Bailey, A. (2010, April 20). Resistance band exercises for seniors. LIVESTRONG.COM; Livestrong.com. https://www.livestrong.com/article/108869-resistance-band-exercises-seniors/

Biddulph, M. (2021, December 10). What are the benefits of resistance bands? Livescience.com. https://www.livescience.com/benefits-of-resistance-bands

Bucci, R. (2020, July 8). The importance of warming up. Www.resultspt.com. https://www.resultspt.com/blog/posts/the-importance-of-warming-up

Capritto, A. (2020, December 11). A low-impact cardio workout for older adults that's easy on the joints. LIVESTRONG.COM. https://www.livestrong.com/article/13730206-quick-low-impact-cardio-workout-seniors/

CDC. (2021, August 6). Facts about falls. Www.cdc.gov. https://www.cdc.gov/falls/facts.html

Centers for Disease Control and Prevention. (2022, April 6). Physical activity for healthy aging. Centers for Disease Control and Prevention. https://www.cdc.gov/physicalactivity/basics/older_adults/index.htm#:~:text=Adults%20aged%2065%20and%20older

Colberg, S. (2017, May 7). Resistance training guidelines for older adults or anyone with reduced mobility. Diabetes Strong. https://diabetesstrong.com/resistance-training-guidelines-for-older-adults-or-anyone-with-reduced-mobility/

Cristol, H. (2021, March 26). How posture changes as you get older. WebMD. https://www.webmd.com/healthy-aging/features/posture-changes-older-adults

Cronkleton, E. (2019, March 22). Balance exercises: 13 moves with instructions. Healthline. https://www.healthline.com/health/exercises-for-balance#exercise-for-seniors

Davis, K. (2022 1). 33 resistance band exercises you can do literally anywhere. Greatist. https://greatist.com/fitness/resistance-band-exercises#legs-and-glutes

Dumbbell & resistance band exercises for seniors. (n.d.). Lifeline. https://www.lifeline.ca/en/resources/dumbbell-and-resistance-band-exercises-for-seniors/

Fancy, L. (2020, March 20). 6 ways for seniors to stay safe while exercising. Home Care Assistance Winnipeg, Manitoba. https://www.homecareassistancewinnipeg.ca/how-can-aging-adults-exercise-safely/

Findley, D. (2022, August 30). Warm-Up exercises for seniors or over 50
• [video and guide]. Over Fifty and Fit. https://overfiftyandfit.com/warm-up-exercises-seniors/

Finlay, L. (2023, March 20). Here's how to choose the right resistance bands and how to use them. Verywell Fit. https://www.verywellfit.com/choosing-and-using-resistance-bands-1229709

Fischer, K. (2022, December 22). What Is Progressive Overload? WebMD. https://www.webmd.com/fitness-exercise/progressive-overload#:~:text=It

Frey, M. (2015, October 7). The benefits of a cool down after exercise. Verywell Fit. https://www.verywellfit.com/what-is-a-cool-down-3495457

Hall, K. (2022, December 16). HIIT for seniors: How to up the intensity of your workouts. Hospital for Special Surgery. https://www.hss.edu/article_hiit-workouts-seniors.asp

Halvarsson, A., Dohrn, I.-M., & Ståhle, A. (2014). Taking balance training for older adults one step further: the rationale for and a description of a proven balance training programme. Clinical Rehabilitation, 29(5), 417–425. https://doi.org/10.1177/0269215514546770

Hamar, B., Coberley, C. R., Pope, J. E., & Rula, E. Y. (2013). Impact of a senior fitness program on measures of physical and emotional health and functioning. Population Health Management, 16(6), 364–372. https://doi.org/10.1089/pop.2012.0111

Healthy eating tips for seniors. (2021, February 23). Www.ncoa.org. https://www.ncoa.org/article/healthy-eating-tips-for-seniors

How to read food and beverage labels. (2022, February 24). National Institute on Aging. https://www.nia.nih.gov/health/how-read-food-and-beverage-labels

How to stay hydrated for better health. (2021, August 23). Www.ncoa.org. https://www.ncoa.org/article/how-to-stay-hydrated-for-better-health

Jeon, H., & Natale, N. (2023, March 28). 30 easy resistance band workouts to sculpt your entire body, according to experts. Prevention. https://www.prevention.com/fitness/workout-clothes-gear/g39590790/resistance-band-exercises/

Kutcher, M. (n.d.-a). Lumbar flexion side stretch technique for seniors | More Life Health. More Life Health - Seniors Health & Fitness. Retrieved August 26, 2023, from https://morelifehealth.com/lumbar-side-flexion-stretch

Kutcher, M. (n.d.-b). The 10 best balance exercises for seniors | More Life Health. More Life Health - Seniors Health & Fitness. https://morelifehealth.com/articles/best-balance-exercises-for-seniors

Kutcher, M. (2019, October 8). How to get strong and stay strong after 60 - The complete guide. More Life Health - Seniors Health & Fitness. https://morelifehealth.com/articles/strength-training-guide#12

Lieberman, D. E., Kistner, T. M., Richard, D., Lee, I-Min., & Baggish, A. L. (2021). The active grandparent hypothesis: Physical activity and the evolution of extended human healthspans and lifespans. Proceedings of the National Academy of Sciences, 118(50), e2107621118. https://doi.org/10.1073/pnas.2107621118

Mansour, S. (2022, July 22). 11 resistance band exercises to work every muscle in the body. TODAY.com. https://www.today.com/health/diet-fitness/resistance-band-exercises-rcna39798

Marcin, A. (2018, July 2). What are the benefits of aerobic exercise? Healthline; Healthline Media. https://www.healthline.com/health/fitness-exercise/benefits-of-aerobic-exercise#benefits

McCoy, J. (2021a, June 18). Try this 20-minute low-impact workout video for full-body strength. SELF. https://www.self.com/gallery/low-impact-full-body-workout

McCoy, J. (2021, October 23). 4 exercises for better posture you can do with just a resistance band. SELF. https://www.self.com/gallery/resistance-band-back-workout

More Health Life Seniors. (2017, July 11). The best stretches for seniors (part 1: Lower body) | More Life Health. Www.youtube.com. https://www.youtube.com/watch?v=J-lH5ksxaRg

More Life Health Seniors. (2020, December 13). Standing stretches for seniors | Full body 6 stretches (8 minutes). Www.youtube.com. https://www.youtube.com/watch?v=4hMWDxZB8WM

National Council On Aging . (2021, August 30). The life-changing benefits of exercise after 60 Ncoa.org. https://ncoa.org/article/the-life-changing-benefits-of-exercise-after-60

Okonkwo, O. (2019, August 9). Regular exercise may slow decline in those at risk of Alzheimer's. Https://Www.apa.org. https://www.apa.org/news/press/releases/2019/08/exercise-decline-alzheimers

Peterson, T. (2017, May 30). Healthspan is more important than lifespan, so why don't more people know about it? | Institute for Public Health | Washington University in St. Louis. Www.publichealth.wustl.edu. https://publichealth.wustl.edu/heatlhspan-is-more-important-than-lifespan-so-why-dont-more-people-know-about-it/

Pinkham, H. (n.d.). 9 reasons to use resistance bands for working out. ProsourceFit. https://www.prosourcefit.com/blogs/news/9-reasons-to-use-resistance-bands-for-working-out

Ponce-Bravo, H., Ponce, C., Feriche, B., & Padial, P. (2015). Influence of two different exercise programs on physical fitness and cognitive performance in active older adults: Functional resistance-band exercises vs. recreational oriented exercises. Journal of Sports Science & Medicine, 14(4), 716–722. https://www.ncbi.nlm.nih.gov/pmc/articles/PMC4657413/

Raman, R. (2017, September 5). How your nutritional needs change as you age. Healthline. https://www.healthline.com/nutrition/nutritional-needs-and-aging#You-Need-More-Calcium-and-Vitamin-D

Resistance band workouts for cardiovascular health: Building a strong heart. (n.d.). Rarp-ID Fitness. https://www.rarp-idfitness.uk/blog/resistance-band-workouts-for-cardiovascular-health-building-a-strong-heart-rarp-id-fitness-blog

Richard, B. (2019). Overview of aging. MSD Manual Consumer Version; MSD Manuals. https://www.msdmanuals.com/home/older-people%E2%80%99s-health-issues/the-aging-body/overview-of-aging

Robinson, L. (2019). Senior exercise and fitness tips. HelpGuide.org. https://www.helpguide.org/articles/healthy-living/exercise-and-fitness-as-you-age.htm

Robinson, L., Segal, J., & Smith, M. (2018). How to start exercising and stick to it: Making exercise an enjoyable part of your everyday life. Helpguide.org. https://www.helpguide.org/articles/healthy-living/how-to-start-exercising-and-stick-to-it.htm

Seguin, R. A., Epping, J. N., M Ed David, Buchner, M., H Rina Bloch, Miriam, E., & Nelson. (2003). Strength training for older adults. https://www.cdc.gov/physicalactivity/downloads/growing_stronger.pdf

Semeco, A. (2021, February 2). How to start exercising: A beginner's guide to working out. Healthline. https://www.healthline.com/nutrition/how-to-start-exercising#1-week-sample-exercise-program

Senior Fitness With Meredith. (2021, September 12). Senior fitness - 10 minute low impact cardio workout | intermediate level w/ stretching at the end. Www.youtube.com. https://www.youtube.com/watch?v=OjQU_f8nJ5I&list=RDCMUC2BaKQ5vqal9yaC-VbpD5ZQ&index=4

Senior Fitness With Meredith. (2022, October 11). Low-impact cardio warm-up for seniors and beginners | 10 min. www.youtube.com. https://youtu.be/7lS1ZwV2Ryg?si=07eNaxlmxFrzSQzf

Six body-balancing exercises that your gym instructor won't teach you! (n.d.). Apollo247. Retrieved August 26, 2023, from https://www.apollo247.com/blog/article/best-balance-exercises-for-body

SMART Goals. (2022). Mind Tools. https://www.mindtools.com/a4wo118/smart-goals

Smith, M. F., Ellmore, M., Middleton, G., Murgatroyd, P. M., & Gee, T. I. (n.d.). Effects of resistance band exercise on vascular activity and fitness in older adults. Core.ac.uk. https://doi.org/10.1055/s-0042-121261

Son, W.-M., & Park, J.-J. (2021). Resistance band exercise training prevents the progression of metabolic syndrome in obese postmenopausal women. Journal of Sports Science and Medicine, 20, 291–299. https://doi.org/10.52082/jssm.2021.291

Stefanacci, R. (2019). Changes in the body with aging. MSD Manual Consumer Version; MSD Manuals. https://www.msdmanuals.com/home/older-people%E2%80%99s-health-issues/the-aging-body/changes-in-the-body-with-aging

Stress and how to reduce it: A guide for older adults. (n.d.). Www.ncoa.org. Retrieved August 29, 2023, from https://www.ncoa.org/article/stress-and-how-to-reduce-it-a-guide-for-older-adults

Ten best upper body bodyweight exercises. (n.d.). PureGym. https://www.puregym.com/blog/10-best-upper-body-bodyweight-exercises/

The importance of balance for seniors. (2019, November 15). Resort Lifestyle Communities. https://rlcommunities.com/blog/the-importance-of-balance-for-seniors/#:~:text=Physical%2520balance%2520is%2520an%2520important

Tinsley, A. (2018, January 29). Talk with your doctor before starting a new exercise. True Fitness. https://shop.truefitness.com/resources/the-importance-of-consulting-with-your-doctor-before-exercising

Volpi, E., Nazemi, R., & Fujita, S. (2004). Muscle tissue changes with aging. Current Opinion in Clinical Nutrition and Metabolic Care, 7(4), 405–410. https://www.ncbi.nlm.nih.gov/pmc/articles/PMC2804956/#:~:text=One%20of%20the%20most%20striking

What is MyPlate? | MyPlate. (2020). Www.myplate.gov; U.S. Department of Agriculture. https://www.myplate.gov/eat-healthy/what-is-myplate

Windom, N. (2022, September 12). Four resistance band exercises to improve strength and balance. Enhance® Magazine. https://hachealthclub.blog/2022/09/12/four-resistance-band-exercises-to-improve-strength-and-balance/

Work your entire body without touching A weight with this 10-minute workout. (2021, December 8). Women's Health. https://www.womenshealthmag.com/fitness/g29565103/best-resistance-band-exercises/

Made in the USA
Monee, IL
11 April 2024

56792021R00129